ESSENTIAL TECHNIQUES

FOR HEALTHCARE MANAGERS

ESSENTIAL TECHNIQUES
FOR HEALTHCARE MANAGERS

Leigh W. Cellucci and Carla Wiggins

AUPHA

Health Administration Press, Chicago
Association of University Programs in Health Administration, VA

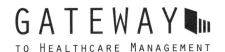

Your board, staff, or clients may also benefit from this book's insight. For more information on quantity discounts, contact the Health Administration Press Marketing Manager at (312) 424-9470.

14   13   12   11   10   5   4   3   2   1

Library of Congress Cataloging-in-Publication Data

Cellucci, Leigh W.
  Essential techniques for healthcare managers / Leigh W. Cellucci and Carla Wiggins.
      p. cm.
  Includes bibliographical references and index.
  ISBN 978-1-56793-335-2
  1. Health services administration. I. Wiggins, Carla. II. Title.
  RA971.C43 2009
  362.1068—dc22
                              2009006136

The paper used in this publication meets the minimum requirements of American National Standard for Information Sciences—Permanence of Paper for Printed Library Materials, ANSI Z39.48-1984. ∞™

Found an error or typo? We want to know! Please email it to hap1@ache.org, and put "Book Error" in the subject line.

For photocopying and copyright information, please contact Copyright Clearance Center at www.copyright.com or (978) 750-8400.

Project manager: Dojna Shearer; Acquisitions editor: Janet Davis; Book designer: Scott Miller

Health Administration Press
A division of the Foundation
   of the American College of
   Healthcare Executives
One North Franklin Street
Suite 1700
Chicago, IL 60606
(312) 424-2800

Association of University Programs
   in Health Administration
2000 14th Street North
Suite 780
Arlington, VA 22201
(703) 894-0940

To my husband, Tony.

—L. W. C.

To the memory of my grandmother, Marie Winkel; to my mother, Rita Grafenstein; and, with all my heart, to Mark Bezik.

—C. W.

CONTENTS

DETAILED CONTENTS

FOREWORD

I am amazed at how, each year, healthcare managers think they have it worse than they did in any other period. We must recognize that the healthcare industry is in a constant state of change and that the application of good management principles will keep us grounded and able to move our organizations and our staff to the next level. As a former hospital administrator and health system executive and now a professor in the field of health administration and a community hospital governing board member, I know that it takes competence, finely tuned professional skills, and great determination to be a success in the field today. Many of my students question whether they have what it takes to be a manager in the volatile world of healthcare with its incremental reform, tight regulation, transparency, continual drive for improvements in quality and patient safety, and personal accountability.

Essential Techniques for Healthcare Managers will allow undergraduate students to begin to understand just what it takes. In an organized format, Drs. Cellucci and Wiggins have created what I consider an important work to introduce a student to healthcare management in a nicely blended combination of conceptual and practical information. Classic management processes are discussed in today's terms, and opportunities for personal development give the student a refreshingly holistic view. The text appeals to the active learner with its definition of terms, thoughtful discussion questions that apply the knowledge gained through the readings, and carefully crafted exercises to test the principles presented in a controlled, safe environment.

Dr. Leigh Cellucci, chair of the Department of Health Administration in the Kasiska College of Health Professions at Idaho State University, has a rich background as a scholar of sociology and brings a unique perspective to the bigger effect managerial processes can have on health disparities. She has worked on issues at various levels, including marketing and strategic planning of local health centers, state reform measures in South Carolina and Idaho, and health access issues for women in India. This, coupled with her academic experience, provides a clear soundboard for how good managerial skills can improve health outcomes and quality of life.

Dr. Carla Wiggins, associate professor at the University of Wisconsin at Milwaukee, complements Dr. Cellucci with her hands-on practical approach in the classroom and in this text. From her background in healthcare finance and as a governing board member of a dynamic regional medical center, Dr. Wiggins shares the critical managerial tools needed as well as her applied experiences with healthcare leadership. She too, with many years in academe, is able to provide information in an easily understood yet interesting way, to engage the reader in the technicalities of healthcare management.

I have had the pleasure of collaborating with these outstanding individuals through our professional association, AUPHA (Association of University Programs in Health Administration), in service, teaching, and joint consultation. I find Drs. Cellucci and Wiggins to be two of the most knowledgeable sources of information on the current state of healthcare management and the most collegial of associates. I am confident that readers of this text, particularly students new to the subject, will recognize the important insight they provide as they embark on their discovery of the *Essential Techniques for Healthcare Managers*.

Louis G. Rubino, PhD, FACHE
Professor and Director of the Health Administration Program at California State University, Northridge

PREFACE

At the 2004 Undergraduate Workshop Meetings of the Association of University Programs in Health Administration, health administration professors discussed in length the need for textbooks that fit our courses and our students. The conversations at that meeting motivated us to write this book.

We didn't want to simply assemble good, timely instruction for beginning healthcare managers; we wanted to create a book that would be pitched perfectly to undergraduate healthcare students, blending theory and practical applications to hold their interest and pique their curiosity. This book is first and foremost a management text that has been fine-tuned to healthcare and to entry-level students of management.

We have been teaching undergraduates for more years than we are willing to acknowledge, and we are intimately familiar with the challenge of adapting text chapters into meaningful lectures and learning activities. We designed our book so that each chapter includes pedagogically sound, tried-and-true teaching techniques, including a running glossary, questions for discussion, and perhaps most importantly, applied learning experiences to illustrate the application of theories discussed in the chapter.

We sincerely hope that our book brings the best of teaching into the healthcare management classroom, for the student and for the professor. We worked to find the ideal balance of theory and application to help students make the cognitive leap from passive reading to active understanding.

In our experience, most of today's college and university faculty did not experience an active and involved student learning process themselves, and they have not been trained to teach this way. The pedagogically sound learning and practice exercises in each chapter in this book allow professors to focus on and delve deeply into each topic and their students' learning experiences rather than adapting, creating, organizing, and implementing untested exercises in the classroom. This allows the professor to maximize the efficient and effective use of time inside and outside the classroom.

Finally, this book has been a labor of love for our vocation: love of teaching, love of learning, and love of our healthcare industry. We truly hope that our book fills the void for a solid, undergraduate healthcare management textbook. And we hope that it "just fits" the need of our academic teaching colleagues who participated in those discussions held back in 2004 and others who echo the sentiment.

INSTRUCTOR RESOURCES

For instructors, we have developed extensive Instructor Resources that include chapter summaries, PowerPoint lecture slides for each chapter, discussion points for end-of-chapter questions, and a test bank. For access to these Instructor Resources, please e-mail hap1@ache.org.

ACKNOWLEDGMENTS

We gratefully acknowledge permission to reprint portions of writings that were originally published elsewhere, including mission statements from Health West, Inc., in Pocatello, Idaho; Kohler Co. in Kohler, Wisconsin; M. D. Anderson in Houston, Texas; and the University of Virginia Medical Center in Charlottesville, Virginia. In addition, we appreciate Portneuf Medical Center's sharing its performance evaluation tool. Further, we are grateful to the American College of Healthcare Executives for permission to reprint their Ethics Self-Assessment and to Harvard Business Publisher for permission to use Kanter's (2001) "Ten Classic Reasons People Resist Change."

Many of the case studies and exercises began as in-class assignments or roundtable discussions at the Association of University Programs in Health Administration conferences and workshops. At these meetings, numerous individuals gave us the benefit of their comments, particularly Keith Benson, Sharon Buchbinder, Diane Duin, Mary Ann Franklin, Leonard Friedman, and Louis Rubino.

Specific end-of-chapter exercises were inspired by conversations we had with our students and peers: Ruby Edgley (Exercise 1.1), Jessica McAleese (Exercise 1.2), Bill Stratton (Exercises 5.1 and 10.2), Tracy Farnsworth and Pat Hermanson (Exercise 5.2), Donna Owens (Exercise 9.1), Suzzie Morris (Exercise 9.2), Leslie Devaud (Exercise 10.1), Stephen Weeg (Exercise 10.2), and Jim Trounson (Exercise 12.2).

Our work on this text has benefited greatly from the collegial support of Suzanne Discenza, Tracy Farnsworth, and Laurie Schorsch. Additionally, Dean Linda Hatzenbuehler deserves special mention. Not only did she offer support and encouragement, she also granted course-release time so that we could complete the work in a timely manner. We also appreciate support and encouragement from Joy Chivers and Suzzie Morris.

Finally, we want to acknowledge Janet Davis, our editor at Health Administration Press. Her support for our project was unwavering. We appreciate her patience and good humor; she became our friend as well as our advisor. Further, we acknowledge and appreciate Dojna Shearer at Health Administration Press for her careful readings of our drafts.

On a personal note, Leigh W. Cellucci thanks her family for their support, especially the children—Vincent, Kimberly, and Robert—thanks for cheering me on. And to my husband Tony, to whom this text is dedicated—thanks with all my heart.

Carla Wiggins wishes to thank Mark for his continuous encouragement and support. His never-wavering belief in her and in all her endeavors makes it all worthwhile.

Leigh W. Cellucci and Carla Wiggins
Pocatello, Idaho
February 2009

HEALTHCARE MANAGEMENT

WHAT IS HEALTH?

Health is an amorphous concept. It has different meanings for different people. It is difficult to measure; one cannot purchase or sell it by the unit. Health cannot be produced in advance and stored until it is needed. In some ways, it is a service; in other ways, it is a product. Still, health managers are in the business of producing and restoring health. As health professionals, we must understand this special—and often expensive—state of being, and our roles and responsibilities in relation to it.

LEARNING OBJECTIVES

After studying this chapter, you will have a basic understanding of

➤ the history of health and disease,

➤ the structure of the U.S. healthcare industry,

➤ payment mechanisms in healthcare, and

➤ the role of the healthcare manager in this chaotic industry.

THE U.S. HEALTHCARE INDUSTRY

Perhaps no other industry is as complicated and convoluted in structure, process, and product as the U.S. healthcare industry. It is made up of diverse public, private, and quasi-public organizations ranging in size from very small (i.e., solo-provider offices) to very large (i.e., integrated health systems such as Kaiser Permanente and Hospital Corporation of America). It is often said that only the nuclear power industry is more heavily regulated than U.S. healthcare. Healthcare organizations act as partners and competitors to one another. Yet within this complex and multifaceted industry, organizations strive to meet their missions and serve their patients, constituents, and communities. How do healthcare managers lead their organizations in this constant state of chaos?

Healthcare managers must have an in-depth understanding of their own organization and its specific set of processes, policies, strategies, and issues. Excellent healthcare managers also need a broad understanding of trends in national and global health, the healthcare industry itself, and payment mechanisms.

TRENDS IN HEALTH

In the 1800s, the leading causes of death were acute, infectious diseases. Epidemics of typhoid, cholera, influenza, and tuberculosis (then called consumption) moved through populations, killing thousands. At the time, there was no general understanding of germ theory. The crowded living conditions, open sewage, contaminated food and water, and overall poor nutrition contributed to the spread of these diseases and death. By the turn of the century, however, public health measures had diminished or eliminated many of these hygiene problems. Improved food quality and nutrition, sewage containment and treatment, and better, less crowded housing led the way. The discovery and use of antibiotics, such as penicillin, in the 1920s appeared to effectively close the door on acute, infectious diseases as the leading cause of death.

In the early 20th century, the prevailing cause of death in industrialized nations shifted away from acute, infectious disease to chronic conditions such as cancer and heart disease. However, the prevailing approach to treatment of all diseases (acute and chronic) remained the same: treatment and alleviation of symptoms. This "one symptom at a time" approach works well with infectious conditions, but it is not effective in chronic disease treatment.

INDUSTRY STRUCTURE

In the early 1900s, hospitals and the role they played in society underwent a drastic change. Prior to the 1920s, hospitals were workhouses, almshouses, and charity wards—primarily places for the poor to die. Affluent people cared for ill family members at home and would not have thought of sending them to disease-infested hospitals. Before germ theory, antibiotics, and effective anesthetics, hospitals could offer ill patients little more than a wait-and-see level of care. Physicians themselves rarely entered hospitals, and their knowledge of health, disease, and healing was limited. Few had attended a medical school of any kind. Many were illiterate, and most had been trained via apprenticeship.

As science evolved and effective treatments and techniques became available, hospitals changed from places of hopelessness, rampant disease, suffering, and death into places of treatment and hope. Medical schools began to affiliate with hospitals, adopting the scientific method and the biomedical model into their curricula. Physician care moved from the "art of medicine" (i.e., watch-and-wait, comforting, palliative care) to the "science of medicine" (i.e., scientifically developed, active treatments and interventions). The hospital had become "the doctor's workshop."

For the most part, the U.S. government did not become involved in healthcare until after World War II. An unexpectedly large number of young men, supposedly in the prime of life, had been unable to enter military service due to health concerns. Not only was this a moral and ethical concern for the nation, it was also a security and economic concern. The government's response in 1946 was to become indirectly involved in the creation and provision of healthcare, primarily through the following three mechanisms:

1. The National Institutes of Health were created to research and work toward cures for common diseases and ailments.

2. Congress passed the Hill-Burton Act, which provided low-interest loans for building community hospitals and clinics.

3. Employer-purchased health insurance was made tax-exempt for employers and employees.

Via these indirect methods, the U.S. government established its role in healthcare. It would not directly deliver healthcare; rather, it would create an environment in which healthcare could be provided to, and accessed by, its citizens.

By the 1960s, the United States had established a network of community hospitals and they had become expensive, high-technology, miracle factories. Real progress was made in symptom alleviation and in understanding disease. Due to these advances and to the incredible success of the public health measures of the nineteenth century, the U.S. population was experiencing increased longevity. However, this meant that U.S. citizens were now suffering and dying from long-term, chronic illnesses such as cancer and coronary disease, which were often still treated as a series of short-term, acute episodes, with the focus on alleviating symptoms.

Chronic diseases are much more difficult to manage than acute diseases. Often attributed to lifestyle, chronic diseases can begin years, and sometimes decades, before symptoms appear. And while medications or surgery can ease the symptoms of chronic disease, these treatments do not truly cure them. Many believe that chronic diseases are never really cured but are sometimes held in abeyance. Prevention and decrease of the incidence of most chronic disease requires lifestyle changes by individuals.

Most people agree that the government should protect the health of its citizens. Most often, this duty is enacted in the enforcement of public health measures such as ensuring the safety of food and water. More controversial, but in the same vein, are laws requiring that all occupants of cars wear seat belts and all motorcycle drivers wear helmets and laws that prohibit smoking in public buildings.

But just how far does the government's duty to protect the health of its citizens extend? Is it the role of the government to protect us from ourselves by outlawing, or at least curtailing, all forms of dangerous behavior? Or is that simply too intrusive? Much of the public policy debate as we entered the last quarter of the twentieth century centered on these questions.

PAYMENT MECHANISMS

By the mid-1900s most employed citizens had health insurance, but two groups visibly lacked access to healthcare: the poor and the elderly. It has been said that a civilization is judged not on how its most affluent live, but on how its least fortunate live. Following its precedent of avoiding direct involvement in the provision of healthcare, in the mid-1960s the U.S. government created two large public health insurance programs: Medicare, a federally funded program to provide health insurance predominantly to the elderly, and Medicaid, a program funded jointly by federal and state governments to provide health insurance to specific categories of the poor. Medicare and Medicaid grew with unexpected and unprecedented speed, and by the late 1970s had become huge, vastly expensive programs. Demographically, U.S. citizens are an aging population, and as a greater proportion near retirement and Medicare age, concern about the viability of the Medicare program is ongoing. Similarly, the increasingly large proportion of state governments' budgets used to fund Medicaid programs and the ability of any state to provide appropriate access to, and quality of, care to its Medicaid population is of grave concern to state legislatures.

Healthcare is a transaction- and personnel-intensive industry. Its personnel are, for the most part, highly educated and well paid. Throughout most of the twentieth century, it was commonly understood that growth in the healthcare sector was good for the country and the economy. However, when the health sector's percentage of the gross national product (GNP) reached double digits in the early 1980s, concerns arose: Was this industry too big and too expensive? Technology was providing unbelievable advances in treatments and even cures, but were its benefits proportional to its huge costs? The U.S. population was aging, and there was no end in sight for the growth of Medicare and Medicaid. An increasing number of uninsured and underinsured citizens had no access to the benefits of our very expensive system. Many areas of the U.S. had an inadequate number of providers. And there was a troubling reemergence of infectious diseases, such as HIV/AIDS, pneumonia, tuberculosis, hantavirus, Ebola, and influenza. These problems led to questions about what role this huge and dynamic industry really played in creating health. Clearly, the U.S. healthcare industry had the tools to restore a person to as healthy a state as possible once she became ill. However, questions arose as to whether it was truly a healthcare industry (i.e., one that created and maintained health), or a disease-care industry.

As industrialized nations moved from nation-specific economies to global economies, fear arose that nations whose health sectors absorbed a large portion of GNP were not going to be globally competitive. Healthcare is a difficult product to measure and assess: It cannot be made in advance and stored for later distribution, it cannot be easily traded with other nations, and it is difficult to measure using traditional cost-benefit analysis.

As the twenty-first century approached, many attempts were made to curb what was seen as the uncontrolled growth of healthcare. Medicare moved away from the relatively loose, traditional, fee-for-service payment system in which providers' payments were determined service-by-service, retroactively (after the service had been provided), for charges that were assumed to be usual, customary, and reasonable (UCR). Instead, it moved to a more rigid prospective payment system called diagnostic-related groups (DRGs), in which a price was set in advance of treatment and did not vary, regardless of the materials and resources used to provide the care.

Another payment mechanism, managed care, also emerged. The concepts underlying managed care were not new. The idea of contracting with specific providers to provide a defined list of services to specific patients, using a prearranged monthly payment or salary, had been used since the late 1800s, when it was the payment mechanism for prepaid group practices. On paper, managed care is an elegant reversal of the perverse incentives that dominated the fee-for-service payment system. Where fee-for-service medicine, in effect, waits for a person to become ill and then treats that person by providing all the care possible, managed care creates the financial incentive to keep each patient healthy in the first place, and then to only provide needed services. Early studies found that managed care patients used less care and had health outcomes equal to or better than those of traditional fee-for service patients.

In actual practice however, managed care did not perform up to its proponents' cost-cutting, money-saving, high-quality-outcomes expectations. Patients disliked being "locked in" to a gatekeeping provider, group of providers, pharmacies, and hospitals. Providers requesting pre-approval for expensive procedures felt medical decisions were being made by nonphysician executives whose only interest was the bottom line. Patients and providers disliked the strict utilization standards and objected strenuously to limited hospital stays that systematically discharged patients "quicker and sicker." Studies were now finding that favorable selection—healthier patients select managed care while sicker patients select traditional fee-for-service plans—played a role in the previous positive findings regarding less care and better health outcomes.

A less rigid care delivery method, preferred provider organizations (PPOs) and point of service (POS) plans, evolved. PPOs and POS plans were a hybrid, combining facets of traditional fee-for-service and managed care. If a patient used a provider from the preferred provider list, he might have a small preset copayment due at the time of service, but he would have no deductible or coinsurance payment. If the patient chose a provider who was not on the preferred provider list, the patient would be subject to traditional cost-sharing mechanisms such as deductibles and coinsurance payments. Providers who were on the list agreed to care for patients using a preset fee schedule in return for the insurer's efforts to direct PPO patients to them. The patient's point of service determined how much that service would cost. If managed care is at one end of a continuum, and traditional fee-for-service is at the other end of the same continuum, PPOs and POSs are near the continuum's center.

Today, a vast number of other hybrid payment mechanisms appear along this continuum. There are as many insurance and reimbursement mechanisms as there are insurance companies and insurance plans. The industry is becoming more and more complex and challenging.

THE TWENTY-FIRST CENTURY AND BEYOND

The healthcare environment remains fragmented. It is a confusing mixture of private and public funding, personnel shortages, and payment issues. In addition, the number of uninsured and underinsured citizens has increased. There is currently no central agency at the federal level that governs U.S. healthcare. Instead, there is a myriad of often-competing agencies with interests in and control over public health programs and the regulation of public and private healthcare entities. Access to services remains dependent on the presence and quality of one's health insurance plan. Even those with health insurance have difficulty accessing care and providers. Our medical technology continues to advance, but our use of information technology lags far behind that of other U.S. industries. Troubling reports such as the Institute of Medicine's *To Err is Human* (2000) and *Crossing the Quality Chasm* (2001) describe a frightening rate of medication and treatment errors and call for a new healthcare paradigm.

THE HEALTHCARE MANAGER

The healthcare manager's job is to create the best possible environment for all health personnel in her organization. This sometimes seems impossible, given the demands and expectations today's health facilities face. Still, an educated healthcare manager who thoroughly understands the healthcare industry, is well versed in management theory, and has the tools to define and accomplish goals can and does make the difference.

Perhaps the biggest challenge of healthcare management today is the lack of time to reflect on the big picture. Still, an understanding of this big picture is essential in positioning organizations and dealing effectively with external and internal threats and opportunities. Intelligent decision making that considers many options, evaluates the implications of each option, and sets a timely and appropriate plan for the future is essential to each organization and, perhaps, to the healthcare industry as a whole.

In 1867, Disraeli said, "Change is inevitable. Change is constant." That certainly remains true for healthcare today. There are new markets to capture, new regulations to meet, new personnel to lead, and new ways to think about competition and sister organizations. The excellent healthcare manager needs the tools to meet these challenges.

PART I

FOUNDATIONS OF EFFECTIVE MANAGEMENT

CHAPTER 1

THE RISE OF SCIENTIFIC MANAGEMENT

CASE STUDY FIRST DAY

Mark Barton entered his new office at Health West, Inc., Clinic in Pocatello, Idaho. He had been recently hired as the communities program coordinator. In this position, he would be responsible for managing public relations and marketing communications, volunteer work, and grant-writing efforts on behalf of six clinics located in different rural towns in southeastern Idaho. Health West, Inc., a federally funded healthcare facility, focuses on the delivery of primary care regardless of patients' ability to pay. Mark was excited to start his job and was thankful that his healthcare management education had prepared him to work in a field that mattered to him personally. He would to be able to help other Idahoans like himself. The patients who went to the clinics paid for healthcare based on their income and ability to pay. When Mark was growing up in rural Idaho, his family was not able to afford healthcare insurance. Clinics like Health West ensured that he and his family received the primary care they needed to stay healthy. Now he would be able to help other families.

Kimberly Lauren entered her new office at Kohler Company in Kohler, Wisconsin. She had been recently hired as a Wellness Program Coordinator. In this position, she would be responsible for a comprehensive and integrated wellness program aimed at improving the health habits and wellness of Kohler Company associates and their dependents. Kohler Co. develops innovative products, such as plumbing fixtures, furniture, tile and stone, and backup power systems. Kohler Co. also develops services through its two luxury resort properties in the United States and Scotland. Kimberly was excited to start her job and was thankful that her undergraduate degree in health education with a minor in business management and her master's degree in public health had prepared her to work in a field that mattered to her personally. She would be able to help workers and their dependents learn about and engage in healthy lifestyles. When Kimberly was growing up, her family encouraged healthy nutrition and exercise. She remembered preparing meals together, playing softball and basketball together, and attending exercise classes together. She looked back on those times with great fondness. Now she would be able to help other families.

Mark and Kimberly are part of a formal discipline that focuses on the delivery of products and services to improve the business performance of an organization. While Mark and Kimberly will work in different environments, both have developed skills and will learn new skills that will help them integrate the work of others to meet the missions and achieve the goals of their respective organizations and ensure that the work is done right and is on target.

Mark sat down at his desk in his office in Idaho; Kimberly sat down at her desk in Wisconsin. Both looked forward to their new management positions and both knew they possessed skills that would help them in these new positions. However, this was their first day of work, and both said to themselves, "Help!"

LEARNING OBJECTIVES

After studying this chapter, you will be able to

➤ define the term *management*,

➤ understand the significance of organizations' mission statements,

➤ understand the function and value of professional associations, and

➤ describe the foundations of scientific management and its application to health-care management research and theory.

1.1 MANAGEMENT THEORY

Management is a formal discipline based on theory and research. Managers acquire knowledge and tools to do their jobs well from theoretical perspectives and research findings. A manager may work in an organization that provides consumer products, consumer services, or both. Regardless of the organization's purpose, a manager works to improve business performance. This is true for manufacturing, service, and healthcare businesses.

In the introductory case study, Kimberly's overall role as a manager at Kohler Co. is in the delivery of innovative and creative products and services. Kohler's mission reads:

> Kohler Co. and each of our more than 31,000 associates have the mission of contributing to a higher level of gracious living for those who are touched by our products and services.
>
> Gracious living is marked by qualities of charm, good taste and generosity of spirit. It is further characterized by self-fulfillment and the enhancement of nature.
>
> We reflect this mission in our work, in our team approach to meeting objectives, and in each of the products and services we provide (Kohler Company 2009).

Kimberly's management activities center on worker wellness programs that will in turn improve business performance regarding the *products and services* and help the company prosper in a complex and competitive business environment.

American College of Healthcare Executives (ACHE)
An international professional society of more than 30,000 healthcare executives who lead hospitals, healthcare systems, and other healthcare organizations. ACHE has over 80 chapters that provide access to networking, education, and career development at the local level. ACHE publishes *Healthcare Executive, Journal of Healthcare Management*, and *Frontiers of Health Services Management*. ACHE also has its own publishing division, Health Administration Press, which published this text.

Medical Group Management Association (MGMA)
A professional association of medical group practice professionals with over 21,500 members who lead and manage over 13,500 organizations. Membership includes administrators, CEOs, physicians in management, board members, and office managers.

Managers in health service organizations create an environment in which high-quality care can be provided. Wherever care is available, someone needs to attend to the business side of the practice so caregivers can spend their time providing care. Management activities need to focus on quality to ensure that departments and offices run as well as possible. Healthcare managers integrate the work of others throughout the organization to ensure the mission is met, the goals are achieved, and the work is done right and is on target.

The managers of M.D. Anderson Cancer Center focus on the delivery of innovative cancer treatment, research, and teaching. The mission of M.D. Anderson Cancer Center reads:

The mission of The University of Texas M. D. Anderson Cancer Center is to eliminate cancer in Texas, the nation, and the world through outstanding programs that integrate patient care, research and prevention, and through education for undergraduate and graduate students, trainees, professionals, employees and the public (University of Texas M. D. Anderson Cancer Center 2009).

The managers of the University of Virginia Medical Center focus on the delivery of innovative patient care, research, and teaching. The mission of the University of Virginia Medical Center reads:

To provide excellence and innovation in the care of patients, the training of health professionals and the creation and sharing of health knowledge (University of Virginia Health System 2006).

In the case study, Mark's overall role as a manager at Health West, Inc. is to focus on the delivery of primary healthcare. The mission of Health West, Inc., reads:

Health West, Inc. is dedicated to providing high quality health care for all, regardless of a patient's ability to pay (Health West, Inc. 2007).

Whether the services are focused on specific healthcare issues or general healthcare concerns, healthcare managers' activities center on improving business performance regarding health services and prospering in a complex and competitive business environment.

Management associations encourage and facilitate the professional development of healthcare managers. For example, the **American College of Healthcare Executives (ACHE), the Medical Group Management Association (MGMA),** and the **Association of University Programs in Health Administration (AUPHA)** all state that their mission is to enhance the profession and promote excellence. The values statements of these organizations also refer to the importance of integrity, continuous learning, and leadership in professional development. MGMA further states that teamwork is important for medical group practice managers.

Theory and research confirm that these factors influence management performance. When managers act with integrity, maintain flexibility and willingness to learn, provide effective leadership, and work with interdisciplinary healthcare teams, employee performance and clinical outcomes tend to be better (Flaherty 1999; Amos, Hu, and Herrick 2005; Lemieux-Charles and McGuire 2006; Black 2008). Therefore, an understanding of the theoretical foundations of management in general and of healthcare management specifically, combined with an understanding of research methods and findings, helps managers to do their jobs well. And, as Mark's and Kimberly's situations illustrate, it answers their call for "help!" as they begin their management careers.

1.2 FOUNDATIONS OF SCIENTIFIC MANAGEMENT

People practiced effective management skills long before **scientific management** emerged as a formal discipline. Julius Caesar kept records of employment and equipment procurements and marked the progress of war campaigns (Caesar 1999). The events Caesar wrote about 2,000 years ago were management activities because his focus was on improving performance (the expansion of Roman rule) and achieving goals to ensure that the work was done right and was on target (transporting equipment, paying soldiers' salaries, etc.).

Dunn (2007) elaborates on the idea that people practiced management before the discipline existed in his discussion of the construction of the Great Wall of China and the Egyptian pyramids. Chinese and Egyptian "managers" planned the projects, organized the workers, and ensured that the work was done right and was on target.

Social, political, and economic events spurred the development of scientific inquiry and the establishment of a formal discipline of management. It is not within the scope of this text to describe in detail the changes in Western civilization that encouraged this development. The following sections provide a brief summary of events from the seventeenth century to the present that shaped our method of intellectual inquiry and management theory.

1.3 EARLY INFLUENCES ON THE DEVELOPMENT OF MANAGEMENT THEORY AND RESEARCH

The Scientific and Industrial revolutions shaped the way research is conducted. The development of the scientific method is central to our understanding of management research. MGMA asserts that teamwork is important for medical group practice managers. Research supports this emphasis. As we will discuss in Chapter 7, collaboration and cooperation by healthcare team members is positively associated with improved healthcare delivery to patients. The scientific revolution influenced the method of research—how the researchers conducted the studies on teamwork. The **scientific method** is as follows:

Association of University Programs in Health Administration (AUPHA)
An international association of more than 500 colleges and universities dedicated to improving health by promoting excellence in healthcare management education. AUPHA provides opportunities for member programs to learn from each other by influencing practice and by promoting the value of healthcare management education. AUPHA publishes *Journal of Healthcare Management Education.*

Scientific management
The study of management activities based upon theory and research.

Industrial Revolution
The shift from an agrarian-based economy to an industrial-based economy in Western countries in the eighteenth and nineteenth centuries. This shift resulted in changes to social and economic organization.

◆ **Idea generation**: Researchers ask a question, such as, "Do healthcare teams affect patient care?"

◆ **Hypothesis formulation**: Researchers propose a possible answer, such as that the presence of effective teamwork positively affects length of stay for geriatric patients following congestive heart failure, and identify measures for healthcare delivery improvement, such as reducing length of patient stay.

◆ **Methodology formulation**: Researchers determine how the research will be conducted. In this case, they could survey team members for subjective opinions regarding teamwork effectiveness and determine a method for measuring length of patient stay, such as reviewing records.

◆ **Data gathering**: In this case, researchers conduct the survey and review the records.

◆ **Data analysis and interpretation**: Researchers analyze the data and debate applications of the findings.

◆ **Data and outcomes reporting**: Researchers present the findings.

◆ **Implications for future research**: The same researchers or others may study this phenomenon again, this time considering a different aspect or implication.

Ettinger (2001) followed this model in an assessment of healthcare delivery to older patients who had experienced congestive heart failure. The findings supported the hypothesis that effective teamwork yielded benefits to patients who had experienced congestive heart failure.

The scientific model evolved from philosophy, sociology, psychology, science, economics, and math. French philosopher and mathematician Rene Descartes (1596–1650) wrote "*cogito ergo sum*," which translates as "I think, therefore I am" (Descartes 1637). Descartes' revolutionary approach underscores the importance of addressing questions via scientifically based methods. Italian scientist Galileo Galilei (1564–1642) used experiments to conduct research. One of his experiments compared the speed of two objects of different weights released from the same height at the same time. Galileo hypothesized that the two objects would fall at the same speed no matter what their individual weights were. Following the method of scientific inquiry, Galileo found evidence to support his hypothesis. French philosopher Francois Voltaire (1694–1778) proposed the rejection of theories that do not withstand the test of facts, stressing the importance of looking "*aux faits*" ("to the facts") for explanations (Voltaire 1762).

Other changes that helped spur the adoption of the **scientific method of inquiry** include the social and economic changes the **Industrial Revolution** helped to bring about. The rise of industry originated in Britain in the eighteenth and nineteenth centuries but moved to

Scientific method of inquiry
The formal process of research. Steps include observation and description, hypothesis formulation, data gathering, data analysis, and findings and conclusion discussion.

other Western nations, such as the United States, in the 1800s. The agrarian economy shifted to an industrial economy. In 1840, about 11 percent of the U.S. population lived in urban areas (Shi and Singh 2001); by 1900, about 40 percent did (Stevens 1971). This demographic shift was accompanied by technological advances that allowed mass production of goods (for example, the Ford Motor Company assembly line, established in the early 1900s), transportation gains via railroad construction, and little government intervention regarding workers' rights. With people working in central locations and goods and services being mass produced, businesses turned their attention to finding rational principles that would make production more efficient and help them to prosper in a growing competitive environment.

Dunn (2007) offers a summary of the theoretical frameworks for organizational management that emerged. Zuckerman, Dowling, and Richardson (2000) discuss current theoretical perspectives (from the 1980s to the present) that address managers' roles. We encourage the reader to refer to these works for a more detailed discussion. However, the main points regarding the rise of management theory that these authors focused on follow.

FREDERICK WINSLOW TAYLOR (1856–1915)

Taylor, an American mechanical engineer, studied efficiencies and applied scientific inquiry to the workplace. According to Peter Drucker (1909–2005), known as the father of modern corporate management, Taylor was "the first man in recorded history who deemed work deserving of systematic observation and study" (Drucker 1974, 181). Taylor introduced time and management studies, during which he would observe and record what the worker did and how long it took the worker to complete each task. Then he would redesign the work so that time and effort were conserved and production efficiency was maximized. Taylor (1911) also proposed four principles of management:

- Develop a science for each element of an individual's work. (This applied scientific methods of study to the workplace.)

- Scientifically select and then train, teach, and develop the worker. (This introduced the concepts of recruitment, retention, and professional development.)

- Cooperate with workers to make certain that work guidelines are followed. (This developed the notion of worker incentives [pay increases] to improve productivity.)

- Divide work and responsibilities between management and workers. Managers plan the work and workers carry out the plan by doing the work.

Taylor's proposals resulted in an increased focus on establishing efficiencies. Ford Motor Company adopted Taylor's time-and-effort approach to hone its assembly lines.

Taylor's work laid the foundation for further ideas about efficiency, recruitment, retention, rewards, and specialization of work tasks at the workplace. Drucker (1974) concludes that Taylor's hope was that laborers could earn a "decent livelihood" through increasing productivity (24).

HENRI FAYOL (1841–1925)

Fayol, a Frenchman who had managed a large coal mining company, proposed that workers should be supervised by a single person charged with managing their work tasks. This notion helped to establish a functional organizational structure for business. Fayol (1916) proposed that the five functions of managers were to plan, organize, command, coordinate activities, and control performance. Over time, these functions have evolved and now read that managers are to plan, organize, lead, and control. These four functions are discussed further in Chapter 2.

FRANK GILBRETH (1868–1924) AND LILLIAN GILBRETH (1878–1972)

Frank Gilbreth worked as a bricklayer, contractor, and management engineer. He knew from experience that money was not the only incentive for laborers. Rather, cooperation from workers was key to bringing about efficiencies in the workplace. Lillian Gilbreth earned her PhD in applied management from Brown University. She integrated psychological perspectives into her consideration of the importance of worker satisfaction in efficiency. The Gilbreths would film the work under study and then offer recommendations for reducing the time and effort spent on tasks. For example, they filmed surgeries and recommended that nurses hand the surgeons the tools they needed as opposed to the surgeons retrieving the tools (Gilbreth 1914, 1916). This change reduced operation time and benefited the caregivers and patients. A key difference between the Gilbreth analyses and Taylor's efforts is that the Gilbreths focused on the workers and the efforts they exerted doing the work. Their motion studies offered recommendations that would reduce worker fatigue.

HENRY GANTT (1861–1919)

Gantt, an American contemporary of Taylor and the Gilbreths, was a mechanical engineer and management consultant. He created the Gantt Chart, a tool that aids the planning and controlling of specific work projects. Drucker (1974) elaborates,

> The Gantt Chart, in which the steps necessary to obtain a final work result are worked out by projecting backward, step by step from end result to actions, their timing and their sequence, though developed during World War I, is still the one tool we have to identify the process needed to accomplish a task, whether making a pair of shoes, landing a man on the moon, or producing an opera (182).

Versions of the Gantt Chart are still used today. Managers have employed the chart to build the Hoover Dam (1931) and plan the U.S. interstate highway project (1956). Gantt's approach allowed for the development of specific tools to help managers get tasks accomplished. With reference to the case study, Mark Barton's responsibilities include volunteer efforts. Mark may design a Gantt Chart like that depicted in Table 1.1.

Volunteer Recruitment Plan, Health West, Inc.

Project—2009	January	February	March	April	Responsible Party
Announcements made and placed in all HW clinics and local newspapers	Start 1-5-09 → End 1-30-09				Mark
Join and present volunteer announcement on Community Calendar on Local Television Stations	Start 1-12-09			End 4-3-09 →	Mark
Appear on Community Channel's noon local talk show		Booked 2-18-09 →			CEO of Health West and Mark
Inquire about church and school newsletters		Start 2-2-09 →	End 3-6-09 →		Jennifer (student intern)
Take current volunteers to lunch; continue regular contact and establish Bring a Friend to Volunteer Initiative	Start 1-23-09			Ongoing →	Mark and Jennifer
Report and assess recruitment efforts with board				4-22-09 →	Mark

TABLE 1.1
Volunteer Recruitment Plan, Health West, January through April, 2009

Max Weber (1864–1920)

Weber, a German sociologist, proposed that bureaucratic coordination of activities marked the Industrial Revolution. Rational principles guide the organization of bureaucracies (Coser 1971). Activity is based upon authority relations, which are characterized by a division of labor, a defined hierarchy, and rules and regulations. Jobs consist of well-defined tasks, authority is based upon workers' position in the organization (e.g., manager, laborer), and people work for salaries and pursue careers within the organizations. However, Weber was concerned about the depersonalization that could result from rationalization and the growth of bureaucracies.

Mary Parker Follett (1868–1933)

Follett, an American social worker and management consultant, addressed the issue of worker and management relations. Negotiation, conflict resolution, and collaboration between worker and manager were central to her writings (Follett 1941).

Chester Barnard (1886–1961)

Barnard, president of New Jersey Bell Telephone Company, focused on the role of the person in an organization. He proposed that the manager's role was to communicate with workers and encourage them to recognize the common goals of the organization and their performance (Barnard 1938).

These contributors to the development of the management field came from various disciplines. Some offered proposals that concerned the structure and function of theory and research (e.g., Descartes, Galileo, Voltaire), others focused on scientific management (e.g., Taylor, the Gilbreths, Gantt), and still others focused on the role of people and their interactions with one another at the workplace (e.g., Follett, Barnard). What they have in common is that their efforts helped lay the foundation for good management and for other contributions to the development of the field.

Management research today is built upon the foundation these early contributors established. Throughout this text, each chapter is introduced with a case study, in which a manager or manger-in-training reaches a decision point. Research specific to the subject of the chapter is discussed and presented throughout to introduce skills, tools, and techniques that may offer guidance. The early contributors to management theory and research set the stage for subsequent efforts that offer substantive information and guidance to new managers such as Mark and Kimberly (from this chapter's case study) so that they may perform well in their careers.

DISCUSSION QUESTIONS

➤ Review the mission statements of the following professional associations: American College of Healthcare Executives, Medical Group Management Association, and Association of University Programs for Health Administration. Identify the common themes. Identify the differences. What advantages do you see for a healthcare manager to be an active member of one or more of these associations?

➤ Max Weber (1864–1920) was skeptical about the consequences of rationalization and growth. He was concerned that organizations could become more depersonalized as a result of bureaucratization. Offer two examples of depersonalization in the healthcare industry. What measures, if any, could effectively address the issue of depersonalized treatment?

EXERCISE 1.1   RESEARCH AND THE CLINIC PHONES

Amy Short is the clinic manager for the Cooper River Women's Clinic, located in southeast Louisiana. The physicians have been receiving a growing number of complaints from their patients that their phone calls are not returned in a timely manner. Dr. Nicholas McCall, the clinic's president, asked Amy to check into the situation, to report back on whether there is a problem, and if there is, to address it effectively. He was concerned that patients thought the office was unresponsive to their healthcare needs.

Amy asked the receptionists who were responsible for calls if they thought there was a problem. They all agreed that they were spending a lot of time on phone calls and returning phone calls. Hannah, a college student who worked in the office part time, said that most of her time was spent on the phone with patients or returning phone calls to patients. "It is not uncommon for me to have three calls come in while I'm on the phone with one patient. By the time I return those calls, other patients have left messages asking me to return their calls. I could spend every minute on the phone with patients. I am not surprised that some of them are concerned about the time it takes me to get back to them. But, Amy," Hannah concluded, "I am doing the best I can!"

Amy had learned about efficiency theory and studies in her college class on organizational behavior for healthcare management. She also knew from her classes on research methodology that she could track the number of phone calls the office received, note the time elapsed since the patient's last appointment, and identify the reasons for the call. She instructed the staff members to document the information from each call. After two weeks, Amy was able to identify the problem, and she presented her data in Table 1.2.

➤ What did Amy identify as the problem?

➤ What recommendations should she make regarding appointment verification, prescription refills, and test results?

TABLE 1.2

Call Log—Results
After Two Weeks

Reasons for the Call	Percent of Total Reasons for the Call
Schedule an appointment	35%
Ask to be reminded of their date and time for a previously scheduled appointment	25%
Ask about their test results	15%
Ask for a prescription to be refilled	15%
Ask for directions to office	10%

EXERCISE 1.2   PATIENT SATISFACTION

Jesse Murray had been working as a patient advocate at Community Hospital for the past two years. He served as a liaison between patients and hospital staff, meeting with each patient or with a patient's family members after the patients had been admitted to the hospital. Jesse loved his job. He was able to talk with the people who used the hospital's services and to improve their stays. He frequently dealt with patient concerns regarding diet ("the food arrived cold") and timely medication distribution ("the nurse took too long to give me my pain shot") and spent time with the patients and their families so they knew they had an advocate during the hospital stay. When Jesse heard about a complaint, he would investigate it and then meet with hospital personnel to try to come to a workable solution. More often than not, a reasonable solution could be found, which increased patient satisfaction.

Recently, Jesse had been hearing patients complain of long wait times in the radiology department. Inpatients reported that they would be wheeled down to X-ray and sit there for hours, waiting for their exam. Jesse met with Rayna Radcliffe, the radiology supervisor, and asked if she had noticed an increase in wait times. Rayna said that they were understaffed in the unit and patient wait times had increased. "But," she added, "I don't think this has anything to do with patient satisfaction. It is just a consequence of staffing."

Jesse decided to assess Rayna's assertion by conducting in-house research. He distributed a survey each day for two weeks to patients who had gone to the radiology department (see Table 1.3 for the survey).

➤ Judging from the survey results, what is the problem in this situation?

➤ What would you recommend that Jesse do?

TABLE 1.3
Patient Satisfaction with Radiology Department Survey Results

	Very Satisfied	Acceptable	Dissatisfied
Length of time waiting in radiology department before you were seen	20 percent	30 percent	50 percent
Time spent with your provider	60 percent	30 percent	10 percent
Technical skills of your provider—thoroughness, carefulness, thoughtfulness	90 percent	10 percent	NA
Personal manner of your provider—courtesy, respect, sensitivity, friendliness	10 percent	10 percent	80 percent
Your time spent in radiology department overall	10 percent	20 percent	70 percent

CHAPTER 2

SKILLS FOR EFFECTIVE MANAGEMENT

CASE STUDY THE NEW PROGRAM

Anna Britton, dietetics manager, jogged around the running track at her place of work, Mercy Midwestern Heart and Vascular Center (MMHVC). While jogging, she thought about the project she would be presenting in two weeks to MMHVC's senior management—Victoria Reynolds, MD, vice president of medical affairs; Lynn Hughes, CEO; Bruce Edwards, CFO; and William King, vice president of clinical services. Anna wanted to launch a new program. It would involve staff from her dietetics department, public relations and marketing, finance, and grounds and maintenance. She also was considering asking the volunteer coordinator, Gail Patrick, to ask some of the regular hospital volunteers if they would like to help with the project. Anna's project would need the support of senior management and MMHVC staff to be successful. She wanted to expand the influence of dietetics outside of MMHVC and build a new, innovative program planting nutrition education in the local elementary schools. She wanted her dietetics team to partner with the Midwestern school system to teach heart-healthy eating habits in all six of the town's elementary schools. Part of each school's grounds would be converted into a garden where the children would plant heart-healthy foods. The school system was supportive of nutrition education and had agreed to reserve a part of its grounds for planting, but it did not have funding to support the endeavor (that is, the schools could not buy the seeds or gardening equipment or pay dietitians to present nutrition classes to accompany the planting, harvesting, and tasting). Anna wanted to persuade senior management to endorse and commit to funding the education sessions, clearing the ground for planting, and providing the seeds and gardening tools.

Anna had been the dietetics manager for MMHVC for 20 years, and her position was much more than a job for her. It was her vocation. She liked her work, and she was committed to communicating the excellence of MMHVC to the community at large. She knew that MMHVC was not only a good place to work, but also a provider of excellent care. When her husband had needed a triple bypass five years before, the heart doctors and clinical staff at MMHVC had performed in an exemplary fashion. The mission of MMHVC is as follows:

> At Mercy Midwestern Heart and Vascular Center, our mission is simple—to treat the heart. To this end, we treat patients with best-practice heart and vascular healthcare, we educate the Midwestern community members about heart and vascular health and disease prevention, and we do so with care and compassion.

The staff members at MMHVC understood the mission and lived it. They had treated her husband with the best medical care she could have asked for, and they had provided that care with kindness and compassion.

Anna completed mile two of her run and slowed her pace for a cool down. She knew she had a solid project plan. She was ready to coordinate with other department managers to develop the project organization. She knew she had the leadership skills to motivate others not only to endorse the project, but to help it be successful. And finally, she knew she had the technical skills to ensure control—she knew how to monitor and evaluate the plan and determine how to get work efforts back on track if needed. Anna decided to walk one more lap around the track and then shower and get ready to return to her office, where she would create a PowerPoint presentation that would demonstrate the excellence of this project to senior management.

After studying this chapter, you will be able to

➤ explain the functions of management,

➤ list and elaborate on management skills, and

➤ understand that management skills may be learned.

Functions of management
The basic responsibilities of a manager, which include planning, organizing, leading, and controlling.

Plan
To devise or create a way to do or accomplish a defined task.

Organize
To coordinate and carry out tasks.

Lead
To be in charge of or responsible for people and/or tasks.

2.1 MANAGEMENT FUNCTIONS

The **functions of management** are to plan, organize, lead, and control. Healthcare organizations focus on the delivery of health services to patients and the community in which they are located. Different healthcare organizations may provide different services, but they all have a set of goals they want to achieve. For example, the managers of MMHVC focus on the delivery of innovative heart and vascular treatment and outreach via education.

Managers **plan**. They define the goals of treatment and education and coordinate staffing, scheduling, marketing, and education to achieve these goals. How well they plan influences how effective they are. In the case study, Anna has planned. She has defined the goal of educating the Midwestern community via the public elementary schools, and if senior management approves her proposal, her focus will turn to staffing, scheduling, and marketing efforts that will involve talent from other departments at MMHVC.

Managers **organize**. They make the schedule, delegate tasks to specific staff members, and follow the established hierarchy and division of labor. Their position affords them the authority to organize the activities needed to accomplish goals. Anna, for instance, decides how quality assurance tasks will be conducted for the community project. The community relations/marketing managers determine the best options for communications between MMHVC and the public regarding the plan. How well these managers organize influences how effective they will be in their positions.

Managers **lead**. They exhibit competence and **integrity**, and they motivate others. How well they lead influences how effective they are in their positions.

Managers **control**. They monitor and evaluate the plan as it unfolds and determine how to get their efforts back on track if needed. How well they control influences how effective they are in their position.

These management functions illustrate what managers are. What they do and accomplish refers to a set of skills. Managers are not born; they are made. People can learn how to plan, organize, lead, and control, beginning with an understanding of the skills they need to carry out their management responsibilities. Katz (1974) proposed that successful managers possess three basic types of skills: conceptual, human, and technical.

2.2 MANAGEMENT SKILLS

Conceptual skills refer to a manager's comprehension of the overall organization and understanding of where it fits within the larger environment. Having a sense of "the big picture"—the ability to identify the interdependent relationships of departments and understand how a change in one area of the organization may affect other areas of the organization—fits into this category. In the case study, Anna has worked at MMHVC for 20 years and understands that the organization's place in the community as an excellent educator on heart and vascular health is a significant factor in its success. Educational efforts have helped establish a long-term relationship between MMHVC and the Midwestern community. Community members know about MMHVC and its excellence in the delivery of education; when they need heart or vascular health services, they know where to turn for excellent healthcare delivery.

Interpersonal skills (often called human skills or people skills) are those related to a manager's ability to work with people. Interpersonal skills include staff motivation, effective communication, and leadership in the achievement of common organizational goals. When Anna first started working at MMHVC as a dietitian, she hesitated to voice her opinions at departmental meetings. She was concerned that her ideas would sound silly and that other dietitians would think less of her. She kept quiet, even though she had good ideas to contribute. Her supervisor during her first years at MMHVC, Lynn Hughes—who is now the CEO—encouraged her to voice her opinions. Lynn told her, "I need to hear all ideas, Anna. I know you have good ideas to share, but I won't be able to consider them unless you are willing to share them with us." In subsequent meetings, she asked for input from each dietitian present so that all contributed to the discussion. Helped by Lynn's calm and supportive manner, Anna eventually learned to speak up and offer her ideas to the rest of the team. Anna had since developed her speaking ability as a result, and she was grateful to Lynn for taking the time to help her develop this skill. She is now comfortable talking and listening to others on a team, an important skill for effective managers.

Technical skills involve the specialized knowledge needed to get the work done. In the case study, Anna does not have the technical expertise to perform cardiac catherizations, but she does possess the technical skills to propose, implement, and evaluate her project

Integrity
Firm adherence to a code of ethics or to a moral code of behavior.

Control
To guide or check; the act of accountability.

Conceptual skills
A manager's comprehension of the overall organization and how it fits within the larger environment.

Interpersonal skills
Those skills that are related to a manager's ability to work with people. Often called human skills or people skills.

Technical skills
Those skills that involve the specialized knowledge needed to get the work done.

plan. These skills include the ability to create a clear and accurate budget for the project, an understanding of any laws regarding the collaboration between MMHVC and the public schools, and the ability to manage her and the team's time effectively to do the job well.

Throughout this text, we endorse Katz's (1974) viewpoint that management skills can be learned. However, there is no one skill set that ensures success. Managing people is complicated, because each person has a unique set of needs and abilities. There is no standardized approach to effective management, but there are tools and techniques that help us become more effective in working with people to meet the missions of healthcare organizations.

The next two chapters address the issues of ethics and diversity at the workplace. We consider it important to present readers with opportunities to understand the effect of ethical behavior on performance. Additionally, we believe readers need to understand that the healthcare workplace is a climate in which differing ideas, abilities, backgrounds, and needs are fostered and individuals of divergent experiences have opportunities to participate and contribute. In Part Two, *Conceptual Techniques for Managers,* we address skills that facilitate an understanding of decision-making processes, the awareness that continuous change is the norm in the healthcare industry, and the knowledge that using interdisciplinary teams in healthcare is the currently accepted best practice—and an appreciation of why this is the case.

Part Three, *Interpersonal Techniques for Managers,* focuses on the people factor. Healthcare managers work with other professionals in the delivery of healthcare. How managers communicate—talk, listen, and write—influences how well they understand what needs to be done and how well they convey the information and address problems that may arise. How managers delegate—assign tasks—influences whether or not they are able to attend to their own responsibilities. How managers direct staff—hire, motivate, evaluate, and terminate employment—affects not only with whom they work, but also important staff morale and retention issues. How managers address conflict and how they lead others are significant factors in their success. Drucker (1988) states that "the leader's first task is to be the trumpet that sounds a clear sound" (14). Integrity is a key factor.

Part Four, *Technical Skills for Managers,* concerns everyday tools for better management. How you manage your time, how you propose and defend your budget, and how much knowledge you have about program assessment and review influence your overall effectiveness. We have included legal issues in this section because healthcare managers should be familiar with healthcare regulations and the law.

DISCUSSION QUESTIONS

➤ Think about Katz's (1974) conceptual, human (interpersonal), and technical skills. Which ones have you mastered? Which ones would you like to improve? Offer examples to illustrate.

➤ How does integrity make healthcare managers more effective?

➤ Pretend that you are Bruce Edwards, CFO of MMHVC. What part of Anna's presentation will you review most closely? What questions will you ask her? Offer two specific questions that a CFO might ask a department manager as she presents her proposal.

EXERCISE 2.1   A FUNCTIONAL MANAGER?

Peter Fisher has worked in the billing department at St. Francis Catholic Hospital for three years. He has been very helpful to geriatric patients and their families. He has been able to communicate with them about their bills, explaining the billing codes and ensuring that they understand what healthcare services they are being billed for. He has also been able to explain insurance regulations regarding Medicare clearly, so patients understand exactly what Medicare will cover and what it will not. Peter is seen as a go-getter and has been able to identify other funding sources for patients in need. His knowledge of healthcare billing processes and procedures and his easygoing, affable style make him popular with and well respected by the patients and other billing staff. Peter cares about the other staff members and always helps them when they need it. He is competent and well liked.

Cathy Schmidt, the billing office manager, called Peter into her office to talk.

Cathy (Manager): Good to see you, Peter. Have a seat.

Peter: Thanks, Cathy. What can I do for you?

Cathy: I asked you to come in to talk about a promotion for you. I am recommending you to serve as the department supervisor after I retire next month. I think you are more than capable of taking my place.

Peter: Thanks, Cathy. I am honored, but I do not have any experience. I have never been a supervisor before, and I have only been here three years. How do you think the older—I mean—how do you think the others who have more experience will take this?

Cathy: Peter, I think they will support you as their supervisor. While they may have worked here longer than you have, you have earned their respect. And, basically, a manager just motivates people. You will be great.

Peter: Cathy, can I think about this for a few days? I'd like to talk with my wife about this and think about whether I really am ready for the responsibility.

➤ Do you think Peter will make a good supervisor? What evidence do you have? Identify Peter's conceptual, interpersonal, and technical skills.

➤ Do you agree with Cathy's comment that "a manager just motivates people"? Why or why not?

➤ If Peter accepts the position, what would you recommend he do regarding his current coworkers? Do you think they will be happy that he got the supervisor job?

EXERCISE 2.2 THE FUNCTIONS OF THE MANAGER IN TERMINATION PROCEEDINGS

In August 2006, the Associated Press reported that RadioShack fired 400 employees via e-mail as part of planned job cuts. The e-mails informed the workers that they were dismissed effective immediately. Derrick D'Souza, a management professor at the University of North Texas, said he had never heard of such a large number of terminated employees being notified electronically. He said that it could be seen as dehumanizing to employees. "If I put myself in their shoes, I'd say, 'Didn't they have a few minutes to tell me?'" D'Souza said.

Ezra Horowitz, the vice president of human resources (HR) at Columbia Metropolitan University Hospital, read the AP report with astonishment. He had never seen anything like this in his 25-year career. When staff members at Columbia Metro had their positions terminated, Ezra had counseled supervisors to meet with the terminated staff member and an HR representative to ensure that the person could ask personnel questions and have some form of support system. He thought it important that each employee be given the news face to face. He even went so far as to set a policy that discouraged any supervisor from dismissing an employee on a Friday afternoon. He would say, "There is no reason to make a termination on the last day of the work week. On Saturday, they might want to call an HR representative and ask questions, such as, 'Will I get another paycheck? Will someone say something "bad" about me to others?'" Ezra said, "They deserve access to answers to their questions, and they deserve to hear the news in person. This is potentially a very stressful time, and we should make every reasonable effort on behalf of the terminated employee."

➤ What is your opinion of the RadioShack firing process? Do you think it is an appropriate method for a mass layoff?

➤ What do you think of Ezra's business practices regarding termination?

➤ If you were a consultant to RadioShack, how would you have recommended the company conduct the layoffs?

CHAPTER 3

ETHICS

THE ETHICS COMMITTEE

"Can you believe this? As if we don't have enough to do, now we have to be on this silly ethics committee?"

"Does anyone know how long this is going to take? I've got a desk full of stuff to do and I don't have time to sit here talking about stuff that has nothing to do with me."

"Well, I don't know about you, but I'm not going to rat on any of my coworkers."

"Whose idea was this anyway?"

"I bet it is just a knee-jerk reaction to that crazy woman who complained that other people had seen the results of her lab work."

"No, I don't think that's it…I think they know that The Joint Commission is coming soon and they need to make it look like we actually pay attention to this kind of stuff. Mark my words—once The Joint Commission comes and goes, this so-called ethics committee will just fade into the background."

"What time was this meeting supposed to start anyway? Who's running this meeting?"

"Well, actually, I am. Sorry I'm a few minutes late. Some of you might not know me yet; I just started a few months ago. I'm the new director of operations. The CEO asked me to chair this committee, and she gave me a few agenda items for us to start with."

"Wait a minute, before we get into that stuff, why are we here? Why us? What do we know about ethics? We aren't experts. I mean we all do the best we can every day, but the job changes every day, and there are no hard and fast rules that are ever going to cover everything."

"Hey, I don't even do patient care. I never touch patients, and I don't think I need to be here."

"So are we going to be talking about professional codes of conduct or philosophy, or how everyone is supposed to be a good person all the time?"

"Well, I think the people who should start thinking about this kind of stuff are the VPs, not us. I mean, whose brilliant idea was it to remodel the radiology department before fixing the entrance to the ER? And how do they think they are going to be able to find a new head nurse for the NICU when they won't pay us what we are worth and work us to death with ridiculous hours? Most of us could earn more working at the mall."

"Yeah, let the folks earning the big bucks and making the big decisions start talking about ethical conduct. Did you hear how much the CEO is earning this year?"

"Well, I don't think that's the kind of thing we are supposed to be talking about. If we're supposed to be fixing ethical problems, we should be talking about those poor people in the LTC center who are just lying around waiting to die. Doesn't anyone care that they don't ever get out of their rooms? My best friend's husband works there, and he says that often the patients don't get their meds on time, and sometimes they don't get them at all! Remember that old lady who died last week and left her life insurance to us? He says she died because she wasn't getting the right meds."

"OK, if you want to talk about things that shouldn't be happening, how about all the lead paint and asbestos in the old hospital wing? And you know that the shielding in the X-ray room isn't actually up to code, don't you?"

"I heard that the janitors just empty all the recycling bins right into the regular garbage dumpsters, so why should we worry about the environment and recycling when they just dump sharps and dirty dressings and the recycling stuff right into the garbage? Doesn't that stuff just end up in the landfill?"

"Sounds like we do have lots to talk about, doesn't it? I understand your concerns, and I know that everyone here is very busy. The CEO asked me to chair this committee because I was on the ethics committee at my last job, and even though it wasn't always easy or fun, we felt that we made a difference. We all face challenges and hard decisions every day. I think having a few basic principles to fall back upon really helps. How should we start?"

LEARNING OBJECTIVES

After studying this chapter, you will be able to

➤ Understand and explain the four-point framework for healthcare managers that includes

- excellence in patient care,
- respect for employees,
- corporate citizenship, and
- the appropriate use of resources and

➤ address the healthcare manager's role in relation to each.

3.1 ETHICS IN THE WORKPLACE

The people in the "dreaded" ethics committee meeting are right about one thing: Everyone in healthcare is busy. Sometimes, in our fast-paced work world, we forget that it helps to sit back and look at the big picture. While each case and each patient have individual needs, problems, and concerns, overarching moral and ethical issues underscore our work and our organizations.

Clinical ethics

The overarching framework of morals and principles that underscores the provision of medical care to patients.

One fallacy about ethics is that it is only for caregivers; another is that ethical discourse is solely the business of philosophers and ethicists. The person in the case study who said that the committee members are not experts and that everyone just does the best they can is missing the point. Each of us must live with the consequences of our actions and decisions. Whether we acknowledge it or not, we each have a framework that we use for making hard decisions about the right thing to do. Often this framework has its foundation in one's profession. Each profession has its own code of ethics and underlying philosophy.

Autonomy

The state of being self-governing. The liberty to rule one's self, free of the controlling influence of others.

We often classify the ethical principles applied to *clinical practice* in terms of rights and duties—the rights every person holds and the duties we have toward others. The four principles that follow certainly do not encompass the entire field of **clinical ethics**, nor are they a conclusive list of ethical principles or acts for healthcare professionals. However, this list of biomedical ethical principles represents those most often seen as pertinent to clinical practice.

1. Respect for persons: Patients' rights to **autonomy**, **truth telling**, **confidentiality**, and **fidelity**

2. **Nonmaleficence**: The duty to do no harm

3. **Beneficence**: A **positive duty** to do good and provide benefit

4. **Justice**: Ensuring that each person gets what he or she deserves

But caregivers are not the only ones who need to think about ethics. Managers and others who do not directly provide patient care also have ethical responsibilities to patients, colleagues, organizations, and society. Winkler and Gruen (2005) propose four ethical principles of **organizational ethics** for health organizations and managers: provide care with compassion, treat employees with respect, act in a public spirit, and spend resources reasonably (109). Slightly reworded, these principles provide the framework for our discussion of healthcare **managerial ethics**: excellence in patient care, respect for employees, **corporate citizenship**, and the appropriate use of **resources**.

3.2 EXCELLENCE IN PATIENT CARE

This first principle mirrors the biomedical ethics principles for clinical practice listed above, yet it goes beyond hands-on patient care to the patient-centered organizational values of "competence, compassion, and trust" (Winkler and Gruen 2005, 112). The committee member who argues that she doesn't touch patients and thus doesn't need to be on the committee has a very narrow view of ethics. Patient care is not the sole domain of caregivers. Management must create an environment of excellent care. One way to do so is to make certain that all hospital employees are qualified and able to meet the criteria and demands of their positions. This is a two-sided coin: Healthcare organizations must be diligent in performing background searches and confirming proof of education and licensure. In addition, health organizations must provide all employees the opportunity to continue their education. The other side of the coin is the organization's duty to have policies and procedures in place to identify, intervene with, and assist impaired or inadequately prepared workers (American College of Healthcare Executives 2006).

Ensuring the confidentiality of health information is another essential component of **competence**, compassion, and **trust**. Confidentiality goes beyond simply following "the laws governing the use and release of information, limiting access to patient information to authorized individuals only" (American College of Healthcare Executives 2004), and extends to providing the organizational resources—including personnel, hardware, software, policies, and procedures—needed to safeguard confidential information. "Society's need for information rarely outweighs the right of patients to confidentiality" (American College of Healthcare Executives 2004).

Truth telling
A positive duty to provide accurate, complete, and honest information at all times as part of respect for persons.

Confidentiality
Holding information as secret and private.

Fidelity
The quality of being faithful, accurate, and steadfast to an ideal, obligation, trust, or duty.

Nonmaleficence
The quality of causing no injury or harm and committing no misconduct or wrongdoing.

Beneficence
An obligation to help and provide benefits to others.

Positive duty
The duty of commission. The requirement to actively and intentionally engage in an action.

Justice
Fairness. Ensuring that one is treated as one deserves.

Organizational ethics
An overarching framework of morals and principles that underscores behavior in organizations.

Managerial ethics
The overarching framework of morals and principles that underscores the oversight and leadership of others and of organizations.

Corporate citizenship
The duty of all businesses to provide a significant net positive contribution to the general good of customers, employees, the community, the environment, and the global community.

Resources
Physical or non-physical features that are present or obtainable for use by an organization or individual.

Competence
Having the skills and abilities to function in a particular way or in a specific situation.

The person on the ethics committee whose best friend's husband talks about poor care in the LTC unit and refers to a specific patient's medication has violated a number of ethical principles. Any discussion of the care of a specific patient is a serious breach of confidentiality. In addition, while we do not know the context of the husband's comments, such an unguarded and potentially harmful disclosure about the organization is disloyal and ethically inappropriate. If the husband truly believes that the care in the LTC unit is negligent, he has an ethical obligation to report his concerns to the appropriate person.

Technology is a double-edged sword; it allows the miracles of organ transplantation, pharmaceutical therapies, and science fiction–like procedures of which our parents and grandparents never dreamed. However, these advances bring difficult decisions regarding length and quality of life. Providing excellent care with compassion, competence, and trust depends on an environment in which patients have the knowledge, the ability, and the right to govern their lives and in which their decisions are respected. Comments about patients lying around waiting to die are callous, insensitive, and uninformed. This committee member is reacting to hearsay and is projecting her own feelings onto these patients. She could not possibly know the life decisions of the patients being talked about.

Since the release of the Institute of Medicine's report *To Err is Human* (2001), health organizations and providers have acknowledged an ethical responsibility to participate in quality improvement (QI). QI is defined as "systematic, data-guided activities designed to bring about immediate improvements in healthcare delivery in particular settings" (Lynn et al. 2007, 666–7). However justified and important, QI endeavors may inadvertently cause harm, waste scarce resources, or affect some individuals unfairly. Health managers must ensure that patient and employee participation in QI is subject to standards of reasonableness and guarantee the confidentiality of those involved, and individuals must be able to opt out if the QI endeavor presents unacceptable risk to themselves.

Last, the healthcare industry is fraught with personnel shortages and budget constraints. Attracting and retaining qualified staff is more and more of a challenge, and severe understaffing can endanger patients. Health leaders must develop and be able to implement workable plans to address "closing units or diverting patients if staff shortages become severe to ensure that patient care is not compromised and high quality care is maintained" (American College of Healthcare Executies 2002).

3.3 Treat Employees with Respect

Businesses should treat their employees as *ends* in themselves, rather than merely as *means* to increasing productivity and profit (Werhane 1985). Employers' duties to employees include but are not limited to fair salaries, safe working conditions, fair rewards and disciplinary actions, a voice in policy and procedure decisions, and protection from discrimination in the workplace (Gilbert 1991; Wynia, Latham, and Kao 1999). Organizations and managers can ensure fair and just treatment of all employees in these areas by having clear, legal, up-to-date policies and procedures on hiring and firing, salaries and raises, grievances, and inappropriate behavior. Creating an ethical culture is a prerequisite for allowing employees to take responsibility for their own actions rather than hiding behind rules and structures (Margolis 2001).

Employees must be treated with respect and justice. Justice means that equals are treated equally and that those who are on different levels are treated differently. This makes sense when you think about it in reference to age. Children of different ages might have different bedtimes, different allowances, different chores, and different curfews. In healthcare, different professions are allowed to perform different treatments, those with different levels of education within a profession are allowed to provide different levels of care, and people in different jobs get paid differently. One committee member commented on the CEO's salary, implying that the "folks making the big bucks" might not be acting ethically. The adage about "walking a mile in someone else's shoes" before judging their actions should be taken seriously before making accusations and judgments about another person's ethical actions.

Health organizations are stressful workplaces. Perhaps it is the life-and-death nature of the work. Perhaps it is the tight budgets. Or perhaps it is the fast pace and the difficulty of meeting all patients' needs and being all things to everyone. Healthcare organizations are composed of a hierarchy of professions and egos, and the associated knowledge and power differentials. Rumor mills flourish. This combines into a highly political stew of coworkers, bosses, decisions, and situations.

Many believe that **organizational politics** is a game that is won by the person who is most skilled in gamesmanship. Mintzberg (1983) defined organizational politics as actions that are inconsistent with accepted organizational norms, designed to promote self-interest, and taken without regard for—and even at the expense of—organizational goals. There is a strong relationship between employee perceptions of organizational politics and high levels of absenteeism, turnover intentions, anxiety, and stress, and low levels of job satisfaction, job performance, and organizational citizenship (Kacmar and Baron 1999).

The detriments of organizational politics can be counterbalanced by fairness (Byrne 2005), valuing teamwork (Valle and Witt 2001), understanding why events at work take place (Sutton and Kahn 1986), and the perception that one can influence decisions and work outcomes (Witt, Andrews, and Kacmar 2000). "Organizations are inherently political arenas and politics is the art of influence.... The trick for managers is to use power effectively for the good of the organization" (Valle 2006).

Perhaps the ultimate demonstration of respect and care for employees is a safe workplace. Employees want to know they will be safe with patients and visitors, other employees, unwanted intruders, and technologies, and physically safe from injuries, as evidenced by the committee member's comment about asbestos and radiation shielding. "It is a basic requirement under the Health and Safety at Work Act of 1974 and an employer's implied

Trust
Reliance on the truthfulness, honesty, and intentions of others.

Organizational politics
Exerting influence on individuals and on the outcomes of situations in an organization to meet one's own purposes, whether positive or negative.

contractual obligation to provide employees with a safe place of work" (Davies 1996, 52). Health organizations have a responsibility to teach employees proper techniques and afford them proper equipment to safeguard themselves. Wiggins and Bowman (2000) found that feelings of safety while working affect not only work satisfaction, but also the life satisfaction of healthcare managers. Healthcare has a predominantly female workforce, and although women and men have similar concerns about safety, women healthcare managers report significantly more actual experience with danger—such as harassment and being accosted by strangers—in the workplace than men (Wiggins 2000).

3.4 CORPORATE CITIZENSHIP

Organizations must be good corporate and community citizens. As participants in a democratic society, organizations have a duty to obey the laws concerning issues such as employment, pollution, taxes, and building codes. Healthcare is one of the most complex, transaction-intense, highly regulated industries in our nation (Wiggins et al. 2006), and as such, health organizations must comply with federal, state, and local laws regarding licensure, privilege to practice, staffing, continuing education, physical plant safety, the safeguarding of information, and disposal of medical waste, to name just a few.

The old idea that "businesses exist to narrow-mindedly pursue profit to the exclusion of all other considerations has been widely challenged.... Society is entitled to expect from business a significant net positive contribution to the general good" (Kitson and Campbell 1996). Today's corporate culture includes responsibility and respect toward staff and customers, help for the broader community, and a responsible approach to the environment (Andriof and McIntosh 2001; Birch 2001; Waddock and Smith 2000). This broadens the corporate focus from strictly increasing the wealth of *stock*holders to also serving the needs of organizational *stake*holders, "such as employees, suppliers, customers, and neighbors in the wider community" (Warburton et al. 2004, 118). Hinckley (2002) suggests that the following words be added to the description of duties for board members and directors regarding increasing profits, "but not at the expense of the environment, human rights, public health or safety, the community, or the dignity of employees" (19).

A 2007 Association of University Programs in Health Administration survey of healthcare administration students found that the primary reason they chose to declare a major in healthcare management as opposed to generic management is the idea of "doing well while doing good." The comment from the committee member about recycling and the landfill illustrates the employee's desire to do the right thing and the frustration that results when he perceives that the organization is not supporting his efforts.

This idea of corporate citizenship seems like a natural for healthcare. Most healthcare organizations—for-profit and not-for-profit—mention caring for others in their mission statements (Wiggins, Hatzenbuehler, and Peterson 2008). Health organizations traditionally fulfill their duty of corporate citizenship via community strengthening activities, such as care for the uninsured, reinvestment of profit into hospital improvements and employees, community health education, staff education, involvement with research, and other community benefits.

3.5 APPROPRIATE USE OF RESOURCES

The perception is widespread that because healthcare services are so expensive, healthcare organizations must be rich. However, due to prospective payment systems, reduced reimbursement from Medicare and Medicaid (Isenberg 2007; Kulesher and Wilder 2008), contractual arrangements with third-party reimbursement systems, expensive equipment, and the steeply rising number of uninsured and underinsured patients, health organizations have tight budgets and must, in a sense, watch every penny.

Today's health organizations have multiple and complex responsibilities; tensions between these responsibilities often result. For example, while caregivers have responsibilities to their patients, health organizations have the responsibility to care for entire patient populations, employees, payers, and stakeholders (Winkler and Gruen 2005). The values, wants, and needs among these groups are often in conflict.

As healthcare becomes more competitive, economic incentives blur. Health organizations must walk the tightrope between financial success and living their mission and values. Some might naively say that there isn't a choice; health organizations must serve patients and stakeholders. However, a more sophisticated understanding of the business of healthcare shows a delicate balance often stated as "no margin, no mission." Take, for example, the committee member's complaint that the radiology department was remodeled before the ER. Radiology is often one of the most profitable services a hospital offers, whereas the ER often loses money. At first glance, it may seem that choosing radiology over the ER is mercenary—expensive new technology for the doctors versus serving people with an immediate and dire need of care. However, the money made by the improved radiology department might be reallocated to other departments, enabling them to provide care that might not have otherwise been possible.

It is also important to remember that money is not an organization's only resource. Health organizations' other resources include employees, time, physical plant, talent, knowledge, skill, and community goodwill. Not only must a health organization use its financial resources wisely, but it must leverage all its resources for the greatest benefit to the organization and stakeholders. Just as the United Negro College Fund's slogan says "a mind is a terrible thing to waste," a talented employee who goes unnoticed and is not allowed to function at her highest level is a terrible waste.

3.6 THE DREADED ETHICS COMMITTEE

Ethical conduct in health organizations flourishes if "leaders encourage and model ethical behavior, reward ethical conduct, discipline unethical conduct, emphasize the fair treatment of employees, and provide forums for discussing ethical problems" (Cropanzano 2003). The formation of the ethics committee, dreaded or not, is one way for the organization in the case study to institutionalize agreed-upon ethical values, policies, and procedures (Giganti 2004). Ethical problems and concerns, such as those voiced in the committee meeting, need to be examined and discussed from a broad ethical perspective before solutions can become institutionalized (Winkler and Gruen 2005).

The four principles of excellence in patient care, respect for employees, corporate citizenship, and the appropriate use of resources raise our awareness of the depth and breadth of ethical responsibilities for health organizations and health managers. Agreement on the principles, however, will not necessarily provide instant conflict resolution among organization members or members of the ethics committee. One would hope that agreement on these principles provides consensus on overarching realms of obligation, and perhaps a framework to guide discussion. Now is the time to start.

DISCUSSION QUESTIONS

➤ Why do you think the people in the case study dread being on the ethics committee? How would you feel if you were appointed to your organization's ethics committee?

➤ If you were the new director of operations, what would your goal be for this first committee meeting? How would you deal with the committee members' comments?

➤ Think about the list of four clinical ethical principles and then about the list of four principles for healthcare managers. Is there any overlap between the two lists? What do the two lists have in common? In what ways are they different?

EXERCISE 3.1   ETHICAL DILEMMAS

Respect for employees is one of the four principles guiding ethical behavior in healthcare management. For each scenario described below, consider this principle as you answer the following questions: (1) Are there any ethical issues presented in the dilemma? If so, what are they? (2) How can the dilemma be resolved in the most effective and ethical manner

Present your assessment to the class for each of the following scenarios:

Mandy is an emergency room nurse who was hired by the hospital two years ago. During her first year of employment, she did an exceptional job. Satisfied patients wrote letters commenting on her excellent care for them and their family members. Her colleagues knew she was a qualified nurse who did her job quietly and competently. Her supervisor noted that she was always willing to come in to work as needed and stated in Mandy's first annual review that she was "an excellent nurse who could be counted on." Additionally, a community benefactor visited the hospital CEO and commented on Mandy's great care of his son in the ER. As a result, Mandy received a significant increase in salary at the end of her first year. She currently earns $60,000. Other nurses in the department earn about $50,000. Everyone had expected Mandy to continue to excel. Unfortunately, Mandy's performance declined after her pay increase, and her work performance is now about average. What should her supervisor do? What, if anything, should be done about her pay?

Sam works at the same hospital. This year, Sam's performance is truly spectacular—just as good as Mandy's was during her first year of work. However, because of the recent economic recession, the hospital does not have additional funds to offer merit pay increases to its employees. Given that Mandy received a large raise for past performance, is this fair to Sam? What should Sam's supervisor do in response to the situation?

Lily also works in the emergency room with Mandy and Sam. Lily has heard that Mandy is being paid considerably more than she is. (In fact, Mandy is earning about $8,000 more than Lily). Lily complains to her supervisor and wants a pay raise in terms of "internal alignment." As she put it, "I just want to be paid fairly in comparison with my colleagues." How should her supervisor respond?

EXERCISE 3.2   RATING ONESELF ON ETHICS

ACHE offers an ethics self-assessment designed to help you identify your ethical strengths and note areas you may want to improve. It is an exercise to help you think about where you stand on the issues. It is not designed to be shared with the others or in class.

The following is from the ACHE website (www.ache.org).

Ethics Self-Assessment

AmericanCollege *of*
HealthcareExecutives
for leaders who care®

Purpose of the Ethics Self-Assessment

Affiliates of the American College of Healthcare Executives agree, as a condition of membership, to abide by ACHE's Code of Ethics. The Code provides an overall standard of conduct and includes specific standards of ethical behavior to guide healthcare executives in their professional relationships.

Based on the Code of Ethics, the Ethics Self-Assessment is intended for your personal use to assist you in thinking about your ethics-related leadership and actions. It should not be returned to ACHE nor should it be used as a tool for evaluating the ethical behavior of others.

The Ethics Self-Assessment can help you identify those areas in which you are on strong ethical ground; areas that you may wish to examine the basis for your responses; and opportunities for further reflection. The Ethics Self-Assessment does not have a scoring mechanism, as we do not believe that ethical behavior can or should be quantified.

How to use this self-assessment

We hope you find this self-assessment thought-provoking and useful as a part of your reflection on applying the ACHE Code of Ethics to your everyday activities. You are to be commended for taking time out of your busy schedule to complete it.

Once you have finished the self-assessment, it is suggested that you review your responses, noting which questions you answered "usually," "occasionally" and "almost never." You may find that in some cases an answer of "usually" is satisfactory, but in other cases such as when answering a question about protecting staff's well-being, an answer of "usually" may raise an ethical red flag.

We are confident that you will uncover few red flags where your responses are not compatible with the ACHE Code of Ethics. For those you may discover, you should use it as an opportunity to enhance your ethical practice and leadership by developing a specific action plan. For example, you may have noted in the self-assessment that you have not used your organization's ethics mechanism to assist you in addressing challenging ethical conflicts. As a result of this insight you might meet with the chair of the ethics committee to better understand the committee's functions, including case consultation activities, and how you might access this resource when future ethical conflicts arise.

We also want you to consider ACHE as a resource when you and your management team are confronted with difficult ethical dilemmas. In the About ACHE area of ache.org, you can access an Ethics Toolkit, a group of practical resources that will help you understand how to integrate ethics into your organization. In addition, you can refer to our regular "Healthcare Management Ethics" column in Healthcare Executive magazine, and you may want to consider attending our annual ethics seminar.

ETHICS SELF-ASSESSMENT

Please check one answer for each of the following questions.

I. LEADERSHIP	Almost Never	Occasionally	Usually	Always	Not Applicable
I take courageous, consistent and appropriate management actions to overcome barriers to achieving my organization's mission.	❑	❑	❑	❑	❑
I place community/patient benefit over my personal gain.	❑	❑	❑	❑	❑
I strive to be a role model for ethical behavior.	❑	❑	❑	❑	❑
I work to ensure that decisions about access to care are based primarily on medical necessity, not only on the ability to pay.	❑	❑	❑	❑	❑
My statements and actions are consistent with professional ethical standards, including the ACHE Code of Ethics.	❑	❑	❑	❑	❑
My statements and actions are honest even when circumstances would allow me to confuse the issues.	❑	❑	❑	❑	❑
I advocate ethical decision making by the board, management team and medical staff.	❑	❑	❑	❑	❑
I use an ethical approach to conflict resolution.	❑	❑	❑	❑	❑
I initiate and encourage discussion of the ethical aspects of management/financial issues.	❑	❑	❑	❑	❑
I initiate and promote discussion of controversial issues affecting community/patient health (e.g., domestic and community violence and decisions near the end of life).	❑	❑	❑	❑	❑
I promptly and candidly explain to internal and external stakeholders negative economic trends and encourage appropriate action.	❑	❑	❑	❑	❑
I use my authority solely to fulfill my responsibilities and not for self-interest or to further the interests of family, friends or associates.	❑	❑	❑	❑	❑
When an ethical conflict confronts my organization or me, I am successful in finding an effective resolution process and ensure it is followed.	❑	❑	❑	❑	❑
I demonstrate respect for my colleagues, superiors and staff.	❑	❑	❑	❑	❑
I demonstrate my organization's vision, mission and value statements in my actions.	❑	❑	❑	❑	❑

ETHICS SELF-ASSESSMENT

	Almost Never	Occasionally	Usually	Always	Not Applicable
I make timely decisions rather than delaying them to avoid difficult or politically risky choices.	❑	❑	❑	❑	❑
I seek the advice of the ethics committee when making ethically challenging decisions.	❑	❑	❑	❑	❑
My personal expense reports are accurate and are only billed to a single organization.	❑	❑	❑	❑	❑
I openly support establishing and monitoring internal mechanisms (e.g., an ethics committee or program) to support ethical decision making.	❑	❑	❑	❑	❑
I thoughtfully consider decisions when making a promise on behalf of the organization to a person or a group of people.	❑	❑	❑	❑	❑

II. RELATIONSHIPS

Community

	Almost Never	Occasionally	Usually	Always	Not Applicable
I promote community health status improvement as a guiding goal of my organization and as a cornerstone of my efforts on behalf of my organization.	❑	❑	❑	❑	❑
I personally devote time to developing solutions to community health problems.	❑	❑	❑	❑	❑
I participate in and encourage my management team to devote personal time to community service.	❑	❑	❑	❑	❑

Patients and Their Families

	Almost Never	Occasionally	Usually	Always	Not Applicable
I use a patient- and family-centered approach to patient care.	❑	❑	❑	❑	❑
I am a patient advocate on both clinical and financial matters.	❑	❑	❑	❑	❑
I ensure equitable treatment of patients regardless of their socioeconomic status, ethnicity or payor category.	❑	❑	❑	❑	❑
I respect the practices and customs of a diverse patient population while maintaining the organization's mission.	❑	❑	❑	❑	❑
I demonstrate through organizational policies and personal actions that overtreatment and undertreatment of patients are unacceptable.	❑	❑	❑	❑	❑

ETHICS SELF-ASSESSMENT

	Almost Never	Occasionally	Usually	Always	Not Applicable
I protect patients' rights to autonomy through access to full, accurate information about their illnesses, treatment options and related costs and benefits.	❏	❏	❏	❏	❏
I promote a patient's right to privacy, including medical record confidentiality, and do not tolerate breaches of this confidentiality.	❏	❏	❏	❏	❏

Board
	Almost Never	Occasionally	Usually	Always	Not Applicable
I have a routine system in place for board members to make full disclosure and reveal potential conflicts of interest.	❏	❏	❏	❏	❏
I ensure that reports to the board, my own or others', appropriately convey risks of decisions or proposed projects.	❏	❏	❏	❏	❏
I work to keep the board focused on ethical issues of importance to the organization, community and other stakeholders.	❏	❏	❏	❏	❏
I keep the board appropriately informed of patient safety and quality indicators.	❏	❏	❏	❏	❏
I promote board discussion of resource allocation issues, particularly those where organizational and community interests may appear to be incompatible.	❏	❏	❏	❏	❏
I keep the board appropriately informed about issues of alleged financial malfeasance, clinical malpractice and potential litigious situations involving employees.	❏	❏	❏	❏	❏

Colleagues and Staff
	Almost Never	Occasionally	Usually	Always	Not Applicable
I foster discussions about ethical concerns when they arise.	❏	❏	❏	❏	❏
I maintain confidences entrusted to me.	❏	❏	❏	❏	❏
I demonstrate through personal actions and organizational policies zero tolerance for any form of staff harassment.	❏	❏	❏	❏	❏
I encourage discussions about and advocate for the implementation of the organization's code of ethics and value statements.	❏	❏	❏	❏	❏
I fulfill the promises I make.	❏	❏	❏	❏	❏
I am respectful of views different from mine.	❏	❏	❏	❏	❏
I am respectful of individuals who differ from me in ethnicity, gender, education or job position.	❏	❏	❏	❏	❏

ETHICS SELF-ASSESSMENT

	Almost Never	Occasionally	Usually	Always	Not Applicable
I convey negative news promptly and openly, not allowing employees or others to be misled.	❏	❏	❏	❏	❏
I expect and hold staff accountable for adherence to our organization's ethical standards (e.g., performance reviews).	❏	❏	❏	❏	❏
I demonstrate that incompetent supervision is not tolerated and make timely decisions regarding marginally performing managers.	❏	❏	❏	❏	❏
I ensure adherence to ethics-related policies and practices affecting patients and staff.	❏	❏	❏	❏	❏
I am sensitive to employees who have ethical concerns and facilitate resolution of these concerns.	❏	❏	❏	❏	❏
I encourage the use of organizational mechanisms (e.g., an ethics committee or program) and other ethics resources to address ethical issues.	❏	❏	❏	❏	❏
I act quickly and decisively when employees are not treated fairly in their relationships with other employees.	❏	❏	❏	❏	❏
I assign staff only to official duties and do not ask them to assist me with work on behalf of my family, friends or associates.	❏	❏	❏	❏	❏
I hold all staff and clinical/business partners accountable for compliance with professional standards, including ethical behavior.	❏	❏	❏	❏	❏

Clinicians

	Almost Never	Occasionally	Usually	Always	Not Applicable
When problems arise with clinical care, I ensure that the problems receive prompt attention and resolution by the responsible parties.	❏	❏	❏	❏	❏
I insist that my organization's clinical practice guidelines are consistent with our vision, mission, value statements and ethical standards of practice.	❏	❏	❏	❏	❏
When practice variations in care suggest quality of care is at stake, I encourage timely actions that serve patients' interests.	❏	❏	❏	❏	❏
I insist that participating clinicians and staff live up to the terms of managed care contracts.	❏	❏	❏	❏	❏
I encourage clinicians to access ethics resources when ethical conflicts occur.	❏	❏	❏	❏	❏

ETHICS SELF-ASSESSMENT

	Almost Never	Occasionally	Usually	Always	Not Applicable
I encourage resource allocation that is equitable, is based on clinical needs and appropriately balances patient needs and organizational/clinical resources.	❏	❏	❏	❏	❏
I expeditiously and forthrightly deal with impaired clinicians and take necessary action when I believe a clinician is not competent to perform his/her clinical duties.	❏	❏	❏	❏	❏
I expect and hold clinicians accountable for adhering to their professional and the organization's ethical practices.	❏	❏	❏	❏	❏
Buyers, Payors and Suppliers I negotiate and expect my management team to negotiate in good faith.	❏	❏	❏	❏	❏
I am mindful of the importance of avoiding even the appearance of wrongdoing, conflict of interest, or interference with free competition.	❏	❏	❏	❏	❏
I personally disclose and expect board members, staff members and clinicians to disclose any possible conflicts of interests before pursuing or entering into relationships with potential business partners.	❏	❏	❏	❏	❏
I promote familiarity and compliance with organizational policies governing relationships with buyers, payors and suppliers.	❏	❏	❏	❏	❏
I set an example for others in my organization by not accepting personal gifts from suppliers.	❏	❏	❏	❏	❏

CHAPTER 4

CULTURAL DIVERSITY

Mr. Khil was an elderly gentleman who arrived at St. Teresa's hospital with pneumonia and breathing difficulties. Admission personnel determined that Mr. Khil could not speak English and offered to arrange for a translator. Mr. Khil's family members refused this offer. His daughter, Seomoon Khil, did speak English, and all communications between the medical staff and Mr. Khil were conducted via Seomoon. The language barrier was not the only difficulty. More than a dozen relatives visited Mr. Khil at the same time. Mr. Khil was in a semiprivate room, and his relatives' presence was disruptive to the staff and to the patient in the room's other bed. Further disruption occurred when Mrs. Khil brought in a rice steamer and hot plate and cooked for Mr. Khil and the visiting family members.

One evening, the hospital floor staff was very busy, as all private and semiprivate rooms were occupied. Mrs. Khil and some relatives were setting up dinner in Mr. Khil's room, and about six other relatives were standing in the hallway. While the nurses could enter other patients' rooms, there was concern about the number of people in and near Mr. Khil's room. Moreover, his roommate's wife could not visit with her husband quietly because of the presence of Mr. Khil's extended family.

On the second night of Mr. Khil's stay, a patient down the hall experienced a cardiopulmonary arrest, requiring a team of providers to rush to her room and begin immediate resuscitative efforts. The code blue team was able to revive the patient but complained to the nursing supervisor that even though their efforts were not hampered by the visitors in the hallway, they were concerned about the number of people in that location. The code blue team captain told the supervisor, "They could have slowed us down, and you know every second counts on a code blue." The nursing supervisor called hospital security to remove the family members from the floor.

The next morning, Buddy LeMacks answered his phone at St. Teresa's Hospital. Buddy was the hospital's vice president for public relations, and he was responsible for all hospital communications with the press. The call was from Vashti Bannock, the local news health reporter who wanted to talk about the recent treatment of Mr. Khil's family.

After studying this chapter, you will be able to

➤ define the concept of *diversity*

➤ understand how diversity relates to the healthcare environment, and

➤ list and discuss the factors of an effective diversity-training program.

4.1 THE CONCEPT AND REALITY OF DIVERSITY

In the case study, Buddy LeMacks has several options for how he may respond to questions about the treatment of the patient's family. He is aware of the situation, and he knows from conversations with the physician and nursing staff that the patient was treated with healthcare best practices. He also thought that the hospital staff might benefit from the Khil situation if they viewed it as a learning experience. The supervisor's call to security was an action that Buddy thought might have been avoidable.

    The medical model of care was focused on the individual patient, and the nursing supervisor who called for security was acting based on standards she knew and understood. She knew that family members should not interfere or potentially interfere in the care of patients. The Khils, however, were acting based upon traditions that they knew and understood. Their healthcare activities were centered on the involvement of the family group and their responsibility to help take care of Mr. Khil.

    Sociologist William Sumner (1840–1910) proposed that people may judge aspects of other cultures based on the standards of their own culture. Further, they may assume that their own culture and way of life are superior to another culture (Sumner 1959). Sumner used the term "**ethnocentrism**" to refer to this way of thinking. Ethnocentrism is functional for groups in that the notion that one's culture is better than another reinforces the culture's belief systems and practices. Thus, ethnocentrism can promote solidarity. (Consider, for example, international sports and the Olympics. Nationalism and patriotism can be

Ethnocentrism
The tendency to judge aspects of other cultures based upon the standards, beliefs, and traditions of one's own culture.

promoted via athletic competitions among the United States and other countries.)

Ethnocentrism may also have negative outcomes. The opinion that "mine is better than yours" can lead to social isolation of groups, which in turn leads to differential access to resources, rights, and privileges. The Tuskegee Syphilis Study illustrates differential access to healthcare treatment (Jones 1981). In 1933, the United States Public Health Service in Alabama conducted a clinical trial to assess the natural progression of syphilis if it were untreated medically. For 40 years, 399 African-American men who had contracted syphilis were not treated, but healthcare provider researchers followed and documented the deterioration of their health status. The men were not told about the study. Instead, the researchers told them that they were being treated for bad blood. *New York Times* reporter Jean Heller (1972) noted that the Tuskegee Experiment was the longest-running nontherapeutic experiment on human beings. The research was assessed by John Heller, director of venereal diseases at the Public Health Service. Jones (1981) interviewed John Heller and quoted him as saying, "The men's status did not warrant ethical debate. They were subjects, not patients; clinical material, not sick people" (179).

The Tuskegee Syphilis Study spurred an ethical debate regarding health research protocol and a debate regarding the treatment of segregated groups in medical studies. In 1997, President Clinton formally apologized for the study and remarked on the nature of the study and how researchers should be directed when working in a diverse culture.

We are constantly working on making breakthroughs in protecting the health of our people and in vanquishing diseases. But all our people must be assured that their rights and dignity will be respected as new drugs, treatments and therapies are tested and used. So I am directing Secretary Shalala to work in partnership with higher education to prepare training materials for medical researchers.... They will help researchers build on core ethical principles of respect for individuals, justice and informed consent, and advise them on how to use these principles effectively in diverse populations.

The outcome for the patient in the case study was obviously not as disastrous as that experienced by the men in the Tuskegee Syphilis Study. However, the incident highlights an example where a family's understanding of appropriate behavior contradicted the hospital staff's way of providing healthcare. The cultural background of the Khil family was not familiar to hospital staff, and the nursing supervisor reacted to the unknown by following customs with which she was familiar and comfortable. She called security, which probably was not the best solution. Buddy LeMacks, the VP for public relations, may opt to use the incident to introduce **cultural relativism** and **cultural adaptability** internally to help train the staff about different cultural behaviors and expectations of patients and their families.

The concept of cultural relativism refers to understanding another culture by its own standards. Healthcare providers' adoption of cultural relativism could improve their awareness of the customs of families such as the Khils. Cultural adaptability refers to the willingness and ability to not only understand cultural differences, but also to work effectively

Cultural relativism
The understanding that another culture needs to be understood based on its own standards, beliefs, and traditions.

Cultural adaptability
The willingness and ability to understand cultural differences and act upon that understanding for cooperative outcomes.

across cultures to enhance the quality of care. Thus, providers and patients from diverse backgrounds may be able to interact more positively to achieve access to care and improve healthcare outcomes (Council on Graduate Medical Education 1998).

4.2 HEALTHCARE PROFESSIONALS AND DIVERSITY

Diversity

A list of characteristics including race, ethnicity, educational level, socioeconomic status, culture, language, religion, disabilities, sexual orientation, age, and gender that indicates an individual's background.

The notion of healthcare providers adopting cultural relativity and cultural adaptability is supported by efforts by the American Medical Association (AMA), the American Academy of Pediatrics (AAP), and professional healthcare administration associations, such as the American College of Healthcare Executives (ACHE), the Association of University Programs in Health Administration (AUPHA), and the Medical Group Management Association (MGMA). The AAP noted that by the year 2020, about 40 percent of school-aged children will be nonwhite. The sheer numbers of racial and ethnic minorities and the resulting cultural **diversity** in the United States have implications for pediatric healthcare providers. The AAP stated the following:

> The health care needs of the pediatric population are influenced by factors relating to culture and ethnicity. Pediatricians must acquire the knowledge and practice skills that will allow them to: recognize and address culture and ethnicity; make valid assessments of clinical findings; and, provide effective patient management (Committee on Pediatric Workforce 2000, 129).

> Shi (2007) defines diversity as differences in a long list of background characteristics that include race, ethnicity, educational level, socioeconomic status, culture, language, religion, disabilities, sexual orientation, age, and gender. What is significant about such a list is that it underscores the differences that are present regarding background characteristics in a culture such as that of the United States. It also stresses that the differences noted have historically separated peoples into different work and social circles. Such separation helped to bring about disparities in access to advancement opportunities (e.g., segregated schools) and healthcare (e.g., segregated hospitals). Because of demographic, socioeconomic, and political changes, people from different cultures are going to school together, working together, and providing and receiving healthcare from one another.

4.3 HEALTHCARE MANAGEMENT, CULTURAL ADAPTABILITY, AND DIVERSITY TRAINING

Let us consider the Khils' experience. The staff may want to address questions such as: "Did the nursing supervisor act appropriately when she called security?" "What actions should the nursing staff have taken during Mr. Khil's stay in the hospital to help accommodate cultural practices yet keep them from interfering with medical care?" "What actions could hospital administration have taken to support the nursing staff and Mr. Khil's family simultaneously?" "What training, if any, could have helped staff members understand the Khils' cultural beliefs and practices so they could provide quality healthcare?"

Such questions address the management of cultural adaptability in the workplace. The ability to understand cultural differences and work effectively across cultures minimizes potential barriers (such as prejudice or negative predetermined beliefs) to providing healthcare. It also maximizes potential advantages, such as better healthcare. Mott (2003) presented initiatives taken by a 210-bed, acute-care, not-for-profit hospital to address diversity issues in its patient population. These initiatives included employee training by various cultural experts, interfaith unity programs to promote better understanding of different religions, public relations efforts to highlight and celebrate diversity internally (e.g., serving ethnic foods in the hospital cafeteria, celebrating Black History Month), and surveying patients directly about the hospital's ability to meet their cultural needs during their stay. Diversity initiatives inform, manage workplace culture, and evaluate patient experiences.

Wentling and Palma-Rivas (1999) assessed factors of effective diversity-training programs. They interviewed 12 diversity experts—researchers who conducted studies about diversity, served as business consultants regarding diversity issues, or were involved with diversity work efforts. All the experts agreed that endorsement and support from top management—the organizational leadership—was essential to training-program success. Other effective factors include the following:

- making diversity training part of the organizational strategic plan,

- ensuring the training met the specific needs of the organization with reference to employees' cultural makeup and population served,

- using qualified trainers, and

- combining the training with other diversity initiatives (Wentling and Palma-Rivas 1999).

Organizational commitment and support by top management is also an essential component of diversity-training success (Gardenswartz and Rowe 2009; Pendry, Driscoll, and Field 2007; Von Bergen, Soper, and Foster 2002).

Dessler (2009) summarized significant components of diversity management initiatives. As previous research indicates, leadership support and endorsement of the importance of cultural adaptability and diversity issues are primary factors in positive outcomes. Dessler's (2009) list of factors includes the following:

- Strong leadership that champions diversity efforts

- Methods to measure success of diversity initiatives, which include employee surveys, employee retention, hiring practices, and focus group discussions

◆ The presence of employee education and training that addresses diversity issues

◆ Integration of employee education and training with other organizational initiatives and practices, such as supervisor appraisal measurement regarding diversity issues

◆ Overall evaluation of diversity management initiatives, including assessment of positive and/or negative effects of initiatives on, for example, employee attitudes

Diversity training initiatives give healthcare professionals the opportunity to learn what diversity is and why it matters. Whitman and Davis (2008) propose that the healthcare management curriculum should promote cultural and linguistic competencies. Exposure to diversity information would better prepare healthcare management students at the undergraduate and graduate level to develop and maintain a culturally competent organization. In the case study, neither Mr. Khil nor his wife spoke English, and the nursing staff members did not speak the Khils' native language. If the language barriers between the staff and the family could have been addressed more effectively, the nursing supervisor may have found another way to handle the perceived problem of the large number of family members visiting at the same time.

Healthcare professionals manage and work with diverse employees and colleagues. Coworkers, supervisors, and subordinates come from diverse backgrounds. Estimates predict that more than half of U.S. citizens will soon be nonwhite (U.S. Census Bureau 2001). As a result, the healthcare workforce is becoming more culturally diverse. Diversity training brings about a better understanding of patient care, but also increases understanding among coworkers.

Healthcare management professional organizations, such as MGMA and ACHE, recognize the growing diversity in the workplace and its effect on healthcare management. MGMA (2009) publishes the following on its website:

The Medical Group Management Association (MGMA) values and respects diversity among its membership. This Association is committed to maintaining a climate in which differing ideas, abilities, backgrounds and needs are fostered with an opportunity for members from divergent experiences to participate and contribute. This open environment assists MGMA in accomplishing its mission by ensuring a wide range of viewpoints and knowledge areas are actively present in our Association and strengthens networking and learning among colleagues. We welcome our members to encompass a full range reflecting variations in race, ethnicity, gender, religion, age, sexual orientation, nationality, disability, geographic location and professional level.

ACHE (2005b) states that:

> ACHE values diversity and initiatives that promote diversity because they can improve the quality of the organization's workforce. ACHE also values and actively promotes diversity in its leaders, affiliates, and staff because diverse participation can serve as a catalyst for improved decision making, increased productivity, and a competitive advantage.

Simply put, diversity refers to the differences among people and their cultural backgrounds. Only 10 percent of countries in the world today have a homogeneous culture (Harris, Moran, and Moran 2004). Consequently, most people (such as those who live in the United States) interact with people of other cultures on a daily basis. Providers, patients, stakeholders, and customers are more likely to work with and treat people with dissimilar backgrounds. Thus, the idea that diversity matters is based upon demographics (the representation of peoples from different cultures and backgrounds), ideology (the lack of representation of people from different backgrounds results in exclusion, lowers access to healthcare, and presents ethical dilemmas), and business practice (the lack of representation is costly in terms of time and effort, and it reduces healthcare quality). Diversity is real. Healthcare managers' effectiveness at work is influenced by whether or not diversity is considered worthy of attention, supported by top management, and a target for continuous improvement in healthcare organizations.

DISCUSSION QUESTIONS

➤ How does the management of diversity help to bring about better patient care?

➤ What does it mean to develop cultural relativism in a healthcare setting?

➤ Discuss how diversity training may influence better working relationships among healthcare professionals.

EXERCISE 4.1   CROSS-CULTURAL LEARNING AND AHA

The Center for Creative Leadership (CCL) is a nonprofit organization focused on leadership development (www.ccl.org). CCL promotes research and writings on different ways leaders can maintain the ability to adjust to new and changing conditions and generate innovative leadership skills. The CCL publication *Developing Cultural Adaptability* encourages readers to think about past experiences in different cultural situations using AHA—assess, hypothesize, and act (Deal and Prince 2003).

For this exercise, think back to a time when you felt amused, embarrassed, or at odds as the result of a cultural misunderstanding. For example, one student recalled an incident that occurred when she traveled overseas. She was touring the Taj Mahal in India, and she had neglected to remove her shoes. She was quickly accosted by several native Indians, who shouted at her and instructed her to remove her shoes immediately. They demonstrated by raising their bare feet upward and reaching to touch her shoes to help remove them. "I was so embarrassed," she recounted. "I was acting very rudely to them, and I didn't mean to be rude."

In the incident that you are recalling, first assess. Try to remember what people said or did. Describe what happened.

Second, hypothesize. Review your description and think about why the incident happened the way it did. Why did the other people respond the way they did? Do you see the incident differently now that you have reviewed it?

The student who visited India said that the incident unfolded the way it did because she had not listened to the guide who had explained the importance of removing one's shoes at sites such as the Taj Mahal. As a result, she behaved in a manner that was disrespectful to their cultural customs. Why did the Indians react the way they did? Her response: "They were trying to get me to take off my shoes! They were upset with me (and rightly so), and they wanted me to follow their customs."

Last, act. Based on your hypothesis regarding why the people involved in your situation behaved the way they did, what other actions might you have taken?

What response do you think you might have received had you behaved differently? The student in India noted that the others probably would not have thought it necessary to confront her if (1) she had listened to the guide and (2) she had taken off her shoes and shown respect. "Instead of looking like the silly American, I wish I had listened to the guide and exhibited better behavior," she concluded.

With reference to your memory, what would you do similarly? Differently?

EXERCISE 4.2   CROSS-CULTURAL LEARNING AND BUDDY LEMACKS

Refer to the case study at the beginning of the chapter. The nursing supervisor's call to security might have been the result of a cultural misunderstanding. What efforts were made to work with the family regarding their cultural needs to collectively administer to the patient and the needs of the hospital staff members to get their work accomplished? Should other people (hospital staff or family members) have been involved prior to security's involvement?

First, assess what happened.

Second, hypothesize. Review your description and think about why the incident happened they way it did. Why did the other people respond the way they did? Do you see the incident differently now that you have reviewed it? Why do you think the incident unfolded the way it did?

Last, act. Based on your hypothesis of why the people behaved the way they did, what other actions might they have taken? What response do you think the family might have received had they and the hospital staff members behaved differently? What actions would you recommend that Buddy take?

You may want to review the Healthcare Management, Cultural Adaptability, and Diversity Training section in this chapter as you think about your recommendations.

PART II

CONCEPTUAL TECHNIQUES FOR MANAGERS

CHAPTER 5

DECISION MAKING

STRANGE BEHAVIOR

Robin Pearhill, RN, MHA, has a problem. One of his student interns is acting strangely, and Robin needs to act swiftly. Robin is the director of patient care at Atlantic Hills Treatment Center, a residential rehabilitation facility that treats adults suffering from alcohol and drug dependency. The center helps addicts and their families begin the recovery process. Robin worked at the center as a staff nurse for 12 years before he was promoted to director of patient care, a position he has held for two years. He is proud to be associated with the physicians, psychologists, counselors, and addiction professionals who understand the recovery process and who provide highly effective treatment in a caring and compassionate manner. The center also employs clinical psychology interns who are working toward PhDs. Robin thoroughly enjoys mentoring these student employees. The students have been accepted by the residents in care, and the staff appreciates their excellent work habits and enthusiasm.

However, Robin is concerned about one of the psychology interns, Jay Brennecke. Jay is one of the brightest interns that the center has employed, but recently he has been coming to work tardy, his notes on the residents have gotten sloppy, and he has been missing appointments. This morning, Robin noticed that Jay came to work with dilated pupils and was exhibiting hyperactive behavior. Robin immediately asked Jay to meet with him in his office, for he is concerned that Jay may have a substance abuse problem. Robin has worked with substance users for years now, and he prides himself on his diagnostic abilities. As a manager, Robin needs to decide what to do about Jay.

After studying this chapter, you will be able to

➤ discuss and apply the decision-making process,

➤ understand the critical role of ethics in decision making, and

➤ improve your decision-making skills.

5.1 THE DECISION-MAKING PROCESS

People make decisions every day. The difference between decisions such as what to wear to work and decisions such as the one Robin Pearhill faces rests in their complexity, their strategic implications, and the **decision-making process** involved. The decision of what to wear reflects the requirements of an organization's dress code and indicates how an individual would like to manage others' impressions (Goffman 1959). Robin's decision-making dilemma is different, as he needs to make a decision in the best interest of the **stakeholders** (i.e., residents, resident families, and the staff of the center) and the facility. For a manager in a healthcare organization, dilemmas like the one Robin is addressing are part of the job.

Herbert Alexander Simon (1977), a Nobel laureate for his research into the decision-making process within organizations, proposes that decision making is "almost synonymous with managing" (Simon 1977, 1). Peter Drucker (1974), management consultant and the "father of management," notes that the "first managerial skill is . . . the making of effective decisions" (465). Simon's and Drucker's writings provided a framework for subsequent understanding of the importance of effective decision making for managers. Recent research confirms their conclusions. Simply put, a manager's value lies in the quality of the decisions she makes (Sutton 2002; Peer and Rakich 1999; Kopeikina 2006).

A manager who makes effective decisions searches for satisfactory solutions to his own problems, taking into consideration how others are solving theirs. To do this, an effective manager follows a rational decision-making model.

Decision-making process
The thought and action that leads one to choose from a set of options.

Stakeholder
An individual, group, or entity that has an interest in organizational success.

5.2 RATIONAL DECISION-MAKING MODEL

There are typically five steps in the rational decision-making model, as illustrated in Figure 5.1.

Identifying the problem correctly is essential to management success. What is the issue at hand? The old adage that a problem well defined is a problem half solved applies to this discussion. Correct identification of the problem may generate ideas for solutions. Drucker proposes that asking the wrong questions is a dangerous misstep, and he illustrates this with reference to the medical profession (Flaherty 1999).

A physician must come to the proper diagnosis before she can approach a patient's problem. She needs to examine the patient, listen to what the patient has to say, refer to research about the symptoms, and rule out various disease alternatives before coming to a diagnosis. An effective physician will get the diagnosis right and can then turn her attention to preventive or curative action. A misdiagnosis may result in an ineffective or even life-threatening outcome. An incorrect identification of the problem leads to inappropriate action, and the problem is not addressed effectively.

Consider Robin's dilemma in the case study. He suspects that Jay is impaired by alcohol and/or drug abuse. Estimates suggest that 15 percent of practicing physicians will become impaired during their careers. For psychologists, impairment is estimated at 5 to 15 percent of practicing professionals (American Psychological Association 2006). As a result, policies have been created to address professional impairment in healthcare facilities, and Atlantic Hills Treatment Center has such a policy. How does Robin determine whether this is indeed the problem? To make the proper diagnosis, he should first talk with Jay. If he still suspects substance abuse after the meeting, Robin should review corporate policy regarding potential staff impairment.

FIGURE 5.1
The Rational
Decision-Making
Process

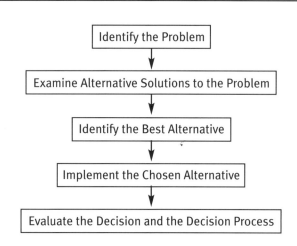

SOURCE: Adapted from Robbins (2000).

When Robin was promoted to director of patient care, he attended a one-day training session conducted by the center's assistant director of human resources. The manual distributed during this training included the policy for impaired employees. Since Jay receives remuneration, he is considered an employee. The policy clearly explains the intervention plan, which was developed by a task force at the center and adopted as policy in 2003. If Robin's suspicions are correct, he already has a recommended course of action to follow. However, proper identification of the problem first requires consultation with Jay.

Robin should listen to Jay's response just as a physician listens to a patient. Communication is such an important managerial skill that this text devotes an entire chapter to it (see Chapter 8). When they meet, Robin asks Jay about his declining work efforts, his hyperactive behavior, and his dilated pupils. At first, Jay avoids the questioning and will not look Robin directly in the eye. But then he begins to talk about his recent professional and personal stresses. He admits to using a drug, but immediately promises that he will not do so again. The outcome is that Robin knows that Jay has violated the center's policy by using an illegal substance. Robin has been able to identify the problem correctly, and as the adage says, it is now a problem half solved.

Examining the alternative solutions to the problem is essential to selecting the best course of action once the problem has been identified. A manager should begin by considering what action has been taken in the past and what actions might be appropriate given the particulars of the problem. Consider a professor who catches a student cheating on an exam. The professor reviews the university's code of **ethics** and policies on cheating. Alternative solutions for the professor may include (1) giving the student no credit on the exam, (2) giving the student an F for the course, (3) reporting the student's behavior to the university's honor code committee, or (4) pretending nothing happened. Having examined the alternative solutions to the problem and having researched policies regarding the behavior, the professor can now identify the best alternative.

At Atlantic Hills Treatment Center, Robin has reviewed the policy and has talked with Jay. His alternatives are (1) following center policies, (2) pretending nothing happened, or (3) individually counseling Jay to prevent him from doing this again. Robin's effectiveness as a manager lies in the quality of his decisions. He knows the corporate policy and is clearly aware of the center's values. Hence, he has the information he needs to identify the best alternative for this situation.

Identifying the best alternative is more than simply selecting one option over another. One should evaluate the possible outcomes of each potential decision. **Risk** and uncertainty accompany any decision. Consider the Atlantic Hills Treatment Center. Robin may consider the effect of reporting Jay's behavior on future residents. There is risk in reporting, because knowledge of an intern's substance abuse problem may discourage potential future residents. However, there is also risk if he does not report it. Discovery of this cover-up could generate doubt about the center's integrity. Thus, future potential residents may decide not to come to the center because of its dishonest reputation.

Ethics
An internalized understanding of how one should behave.

Risk
Uncertainty in an outcome.

Robin should also consider the critical factor of ethics. As Drucker (1967) asserts, "one has to start out with what is right rather than what is acceptable" (134). "Business ethics" is not an oxymoron. The decision-making process should include an evaluation of professional codes and corporate policy and an examination of the interests of those who hold a stake in the outcome (Hartman 1998). Robin should not only examine corporate policy, he should also consider the interests of the residents, their families, and the staff members.

Robin is an employee of the center, and any decision he makes reflects on the organization and its responsibilities to residents. Caplow (1983) notes that a manager of a stable organization is more representative than initiative and that his success is measured by how well the constituents' wishes are followed. Robin knows that the task force who wrote the corporate policy regarding impaired staff had followed a democratic process that included stakeholder input and well-researched action plans. Thus, he determines that the best alternative is to follow this corporate policy.

Implementing the chosen alternative is essential once the best course of action has been determined. The center policy for impaired staff calls for Jay's placement on a leave of absence from his work responsibilities. He may take his accrued sick leave, and the center will pay for evaluation and treatment costs that are not covered by Jay's health insurance. Jay's counseling and drug treatment are to be overseen by one of the center's staff psychologists, and depending upon the psychologist's reports and the staff team members' assessment of Jay's progress, Jay may resume his duties after three to six months. To ensure stability, there is a process to replace any team member who must exit the team.

The result is that Jay has an opportunity to address his addiction issues, recover, and work again in the future. However, his progress toward his PhD is delayed, and his future as a professional clinical psychologist is no longer certain. Nonetheless, Robin's decision to follow the corporate policy and implement the chosen alternative ensures that the stakeholders' wishes are followed, and his decision is in the best interest of the facility and residents. Robin notifies the human resources director, who then takes over as plan implementation leader and chair of the team that will follow Jay's progress.

Caplow (1983) states that the main factors for managing a stable organization include the following:

1. adherence to traditional procedures;

2. slow-moving, intensive problem-solving efforts;

3. democratic participation in decision making;

4. meticulous and accessible records and accounts; and

5. a system for the designation of successors designed to prevent surprises.

Robin followed traditional procedures by selecting the best alternative from among those he identified. The HR director, Robin, and the monitoring psychologist will follow the problem-solving efforts on behalf of Jay (his recovery) and the institution (the stakeholders' wishes were followed, and employee impairment was identified and addressed before any stakeholder was harmed). In this case, the democratic decision making rests with the task force that wrote the professional impairment policy and the team that will follow Jay's rehabilitation process. This latter team will decide whether or not to reinstate Jay. They will create meticulous records to ensure that the center's policies are followed before they assess Jay's ability to return to work. The team will designate successors to follow Jay's progress and prevent any surprises.

Evaluating the decision and the decision process ensures that the problem was identified correctly and assesses whether the plan implemented addressed the problem appropriately. For Robin, the problem was that an employee was impaired. The plan implemented was to follow the corporate policy and procedures regarding an impaired professional. The team that follows Jay's recovery should assess his progress and the appropriateness of the impaired professional policies. Can the policy be improved? Is the timeframe indicated (three to six months) appropriate for recovery? How much supervision should Jay have if he returns to work? Should all staff be tested for drugs? Evaluating the decision and the decision process may help to ensure that the institution's needs and the stakeholders' wishes are met effectively as problems are identified and addressed within an organization.

Why did Robin follow this rational decision-making process when the center had a policy regarding suspected employee drug use? Fortunately for Robin, the center is stable and prepared to address the presence of an impaired professional. Robin also had support and guidance from the director of the human resources department. However, not all managers have the support Robin enjoys at work. The rational decision-making model is particularly valuable where a stable system is not in place.

Consider the situation of Sherron Watkins, once the vice president of corporate development at Enron. Today, Watkins is known as the "Enron whistle-blower." She became suspicious of wrongdoing when she analyzed certain assets Enron expected to sell and determined that Enron was using its own stock to post a gain or loss on its income statement, which is prohibited by the United States' Generally Accepted Accounting Principles (GAAP). Concerned that she would lose her job if she confronted her direct supervisor, she reported her concerns to Ken Lay, CEO of Enron. In court, Watkins testified that her supervisor did want her "out of Enron" after he learned of her meeting with Lay (United Press International 2002). Given the obstacles Watkins faced and her concern for her livelihood, why did she make the decision to confront Lay? Watkins wrote in her memo to Lay that her personal history and who she was spurred her action. She had worked for Enron for eight years, and her work efforts would mean nothing on her resume, given Enron's current condition. Thus, her decision making followed a decision-making model, but without the support that Robin had.

5.3 IMPROVING DECISION-MAKING SKILLS

Communicating effectively is essential in identifying a problem and gathering the facts and relevant information. Consider Robin's dilemma. What if Jay had explained that his pupils were dilated from an eye exam, and had shown Robin his appointment card? This explanation addresses Robin's concerns. However, Jay's explanation does not address his declining work performance. Robin needs to listen closely to Jay's explanation for why his work efforts have slowed. He needs to avoid distractions, such as answering the phone or reading his mail. Open, positive, nonverbal communication, such as looking at Jay as he speaks and encouraging him to continue, will aid Robin in the process (Hensel 2000; Ruusuvuori 2001). Finally, summarizing what Jay has told him will help Robin ensure that he has heard correctly and may help him determine whether there is an impairment problem.

Avoiding **bias** is also important. Through the process of socialization, an individual acquires a self-identity and **internalizes** (to a degree) a cognitive frame of reference for interpersonal relations and a moral conscience (Parsons 1951). Parents, other family members, teachers, colleagues, bosses, and others play a role in this lifelong process. Reutter and colleagues (1997) examined student nurses and the role of socialization on their learning. The **socialization process** in nursing school helps to ensure that the students internalize the nursing profession's values, norms, and behaviors. We not only internalize the values, norms, and behaviors associated with our culture as a consequence of the socialization process, but we also internalize biases, often based on gender, race, religion, socioeconomic status, or other cultural designations. Recognizing our biases enables us to understand that they influence our decisions. This awareness improves our ability to make decisions.

Recognizing a programmed decision and being able to differentiate it from a **nonprogrammed decision** is important for managers approaching a potential problem. Programmed decisions are routine and recurring. For example, Robin regularly makes decisions regarding daily operations activities for the residents. Decisions regarding supplies for the residents' rooms and room assignments for individual and group therapy sessions are examples of programmed decisions because they are frequent, routine decisions needed for operational activities. Nonprogrammed decisions address unusual problems. Robin's decision regarding Jay was nonprogrammed because there is nothing recurring or routine about Jay's behavior. Hence, while the center had a policy regarding impaired professionals, addressing the issue as nonprogrammed was in the best interest of the institution and its stakeholders because it involved a staff member who could have harmed a resident or a staff member, hurt the center's reputation, and hurt himself.

Being timely is significant because even the best decisions are not helpful if they are made too late. Robin immediately removed Jay from working with patients and met with him to discuss his concerns. He did not wait to initiate action until he had gathered more information or talked with others. Had he waited, Jay might have caused harm. Timely response to problems is essential to effective decision making.

Bias

A tendency to apply a negative or positive bent to a situation because of prejudicial thought.

Internalize

To incorporate values, beliefs, or norms as self-guiding principles.

Socialization process

The process whereby people learn values, beliefs, and norms.

Nonprogrammed decision

A decision for which there is no set procedure in place, and that must be resolved via rational thinking and action.

Making assurances one can keep builds trust. A manager may promise pay raises to generate a temporary positive response, even though she does not have the authority to ensure that the raises are given. However, promising only what one can deliver develops professional trust based on honesty. Robin did not promise Jay that his work would continue as usual. Rather, he met with Jay and communicated his concern about Jay's behavior. He expressed concern instead of making promises he could not keep.

Creativity in a rational decision-making process should be supported. Brainstorming alternative solutions to a problem allows for expansion on standard, conventional approaches to problem solving. Creative thinking may generate innovative, appropriate solutions.

Including an ethical checklist will ensure better decision making. Managers' positions make them more visible and give them higher levels of responsibility in the organization. Therefore, viewing ethics as an essential factor in effective management decisions recognizes that managers should consider their role as one of responsibility. Drucker (2001) proposes that managers should observe the ethics of responsibility. It is the manager's responsibility to consider the needs of the stakeholders and of the institution and to decide what is right. Ross, Wenzel, and Mitlyng (2002) discuss ethics and values as personal healthcare leadership competencies. They refer to Nash's (1989) list of questions designed for ethical guidance. Answering the following questions may reaffirm the manager's decision regarding the problem, if he is content with the answers:

1. Have you accurately defined the problem?

2. How would you define the problem if you stood on the other side of the fence?

3. How did this situation occur in the first place?

4. To whom and to what do you give your loyalty as a person and as a member of the corporation?

5. What is your intention in making this decision?

6. How does this intention compare with the probable results?

7. Whom could your decision or action injure?

8. Can you discuss the decision with the affected parties before making the decision?

9. Are you confident that your decision will be as valid over a long period of time as it seems now?

10. Could you discuss without qualm your decision or action to your boss, your CEO, the board of directors, your family, and society as a whole?

11. What is the symbolic potential of your action, if understood? If misunderstood?

12. Under what conditions would you allow exceptions to your stand? (Ross, Wenzel, and Mitlyng 2002, 133–4)

How do you think Robin at the Atlantic Hills Treatment Center would answer these questions? Do you think he would be at ease with his answers?

DISCUSSION QUESTIONS

➤ Evaluate this statement: The value of a manager lies in the quality of the decisions she makes. Consider an example from your own work experience that illustrates the importance of quality decisions.

➤ An old adage says that once a problem has been correctly identified, it is half solved. What would be the ramifications of Robin's misidentifying a problem in the case study?

➤ Why would one want to generate several alternative solutions to a problem? What is the role of creativity in the process?

EXERCISE 5.1   "WHAT DO WE DO ABOUT JOE?"

Joe, a nurse, is outgoing, energetic, and athletic. He enjoys telling stories about his cross-country ski races. However, his talkative nature bothered Sue, the nursing manager of the operating room. Sue noticed that the whole surgical nursing team would stop and encourage Joe to continue telling his racing stories. It didn't seem to interfere with surgery or daily work tasks, but Sue was concerned because it didn't seem to bother Joe that he was doing it during working hours or that someone other than his coworkers might be listening. Joe seemed to just enjoy being in the spotlight, and the other nurses enjoyed his stories. Joe's nursing team performed extremely well. The surgeries went smoothly, and the surgeons often directed that Joe's nursing team assist their scheduled surgeries. From the surgeons' perspective, this nursing team made certain that all was ready and that few, if any, errors were made. But the frequent storytelling breaks bothered the OR supervisor. Sue believed that Joe's team was setting a bad example for the other nursing teams and the rest of the nursing staff.

Sue had just recently taken charge of the surgical ward, and she was determined to do her job well. She thought she could point out to Joe that his behavior was inappropriate, and he would change. Additionally, she knew that she could tell the other nurses that they should not be listening to Joe's nonsense. Sue called Joe in to discuss the situation. She told Joe that he and his colleagues could make better use of their time. Joe promised that he would try.

Things did improve, but after a few weeks, the old pattern reemerged. Sue then met with the other members of the nursing team individually. However, the nursing team maintained their habits, and Sue was left to ponder what to do about Joe.

➤ What is the problem in this case?
➤ What options do you see to address the problem?
➤ What do you recommend and why?

EXERCISE 5.2   WHEN TWO HOSPITALS BECOME ONE

Margaret Rheinhart is a marketing representative in the public relations department at Holy Cross Community Hospital in rural Wyoming. Holy Cross is a nonprofit hospital based on the Catholic principle of providing compassionate care to anyone who needs it. Holy Cross is taking over the for-profit Roper Hospital. Roper's profits have not met its administration's estimates, and Roper is divesting its interests in all of its rural locations in the Northwest this month. As a result of the merger, Holy Cross will now be the only hospital in the community. Other primary care clinics exist in the area; however, Holy Cross will be the only facility within 50 miles to provide medical attention that requires an overnight stay.

The original hospital sites were only five miles apart, so hospital operations will be divided between the two sites. Administrators will stay on one campus, and clinic and patient care will reside at the other site. Thus, the newly formed Holy Cross Hospital does not need all the staff members who had been employed by the two separate facilities. All employees will reapply to the new Holy Cross, and interviews will be held next month. The new Holy Cross hopes to have its new staff—the best of the old Holy Cross and Roper—together within 90 days after interviews have been completed. Holy Cross employees who are not rehired will receive a 90-day severance package.

Margaret enjoys her job as the marketing representative in public relations at Holy Cross, but she is one of the many employees who must now reapply for the position. She knows that Luca Browning, the marketing representative from Roper, wants to stay in the community and will also be applying. Margaret knows that Luca is qualified. He has an undergraduate degree in marketing and has been taking online courses toward a masters in healthcare administration. He has been working in public relations at Roper for two years. Margaret has a nursing degree, and after an ATV accident five years ago, she found her injuries made the physical demands of being a floor nurse impossible. During her recovery time, the public relations director needed a marketing representative, and the CEO of Holy Cross knew that Margaret was a quick learner. Margaret has done an excellent job during her four and a half years in the position. While her degree is not in marketing, she knows she has the experience to be an effective marketing representative for the new Holy Cross.

Margaret knows that Luca has a secret. He has a computer, printer, and fax machine at his home that had belonged to Roper. She saw it in his house six months ago. Additionally, she knows he uses his Roper work cell phone for personal calls. Margaret wonders if she should tell HR at Holy Cross what she knows about Luca.

➤ Using Nash's (1989) list of questions designed for ethical guidance, evaluate Margaret's dilemma.
➤ What personal issues may influence Margaret's decision?
➤ What course of action do you recommend for Margaret?

CHAPTER 6

CHANGE IS CONSTANT

Alfred Lockhart needed to get Mariana Buchanan on board. But how could he convince this "old-timer" it was time to change? Alfred had been the business manager at the Wasatch Primary Healthcare Clinics (WPHC), a consortium of three clinics that serve five counties in Utah, for nine months. WPHC had hired him as soon as he had earned his MBA with an emphasis in healthcare management, and the clinic physicians had encouraged him to introduce efficient office management protocols to their three clinics. Changing reimbursement schedules of insurance contracts and rising operation costs had sent them in search of ways to cut costs without a negative effect on current operations. Some of the physicians advocated purchasing new equipment; others wanted to raise the clinic staff's salaries. All of the physicians agreed that Alfred's efficiency measures should align with their clinic mission: Be responsible to the patient, be responsible to the staff, and provide excellent primary care for the people of Utah. Alfred had started his job with enthusiasm and confidence that he could help create efficiencies that achieved the physicians' vision of keeping pace with technology and raising staff salaries.

Once Alfred had set up office, he personally met with the three clinic office managers. He told them he was there to improve the clinics and would be informing them of changes that would bring this about. He was surprised that the managers had asked few questions, but he assumed that they were on board and in agreement with him. He followed up with them via e-mail, instructing the managers to meet as a group every two weeks to move forward with his assignments. Alfred had not attended any of these meetings.

To date, none of his recommendations had been implemented. He knew that one of the office managers, Mariana Buchanan, had been negative about his ideas. In fact, she had often called the other two office managers to complain about him and his efficiency plan. One of these office managers had met with Alfred to express her concern about the situation. The office manager explained, "Mariana is starting to get on my nerves. Every time we office managers get together, she just complains all the time. I am beginning to dread talking with her."

Mariana had earned an associate's degree in medical assisting 15 years ago, and she had been a clinic office manager for over 20 years. She liked to run the office the way she had been taught at the local university. "If it isn't broken, don't fix it" was her motto. She knew that Alfred's plan was designed to make the offices more efficient, but she did not understand why he wanted to change everything she had been doing for many years. He had never asked for her opinion, even though she had a lot of experience and on-the-job training. Furthermore, she knew what worked. She was exasperated by his decision that the clinic needed a central patient database. What was wrong with the current system, in which each clinic followed its own protocol regarding patient files? Why change what works?

After studying this chapter, you will be able to

➤ define and illustrate the concepts of unexpected and managed change,

➤ outline the process of managed changed from decision-making through implementation,

➤ understand resistance to change, and

➤ apply methods for addressing resistance to change.

6.1 GENERAL CHANGE AND MANAGED CHANGE

The introduction to this text presented the concept that change is constant in the healthcare industry. Sometimes the change is unexpected. For example, Hurricane Katrina arrived in New Orleans in August of 2005. The Category 5 hurricane caused the levee system to fail, and the resulting flooding yielded waters as high as 13 feet through much of midtown and New Orleans East. The patients and remaining staff at Charity Hospital experienced a loss of electrical power and a lack of food and water, and few medications were available. They offered medical care to 250 patients in these conditions while waiting for help to arrive (Sternberg 2002). It took almost six days to evacuate all patients and staff, and the hospital staff's efforts during that time have been described as heroic (Emergency Medicine Residents Association 2007). The situation at Charity Hospital is an example of change that happened *to* a healthcare organization. Most of the change a manager confronts is managed change. In managed change, people in the organization are working to effect changes that have been determined to fit with the organizational mission and purpose and make the organization better.

The change confronting Alfred Lockhart at the Wasatch Primary Healthcare Clinics is managed change. He is trying to initiate change designed to help the clinics become better and more efficient. However, he is experiencing resistance.

Managers lead changes that are:

1. procedures designed for efficiency (such as Alfred's plan),

2. responses to identified problems at the workplace,

3. actions to improve healthcare delivery,

4. adaptations to environmental and/or technical changes that have occurred outside the organization, and

5. responses to ensure a good fit with the organizational mission.

For example, technological advancement in medical imaging effects a change in hiring practice so that the organization may hire and keep radiological technicians who can use the new technology properly. Furthermore, managers lead change efforts to help the healthcare facility become better able to meet its mission and strategic goals (Jick 1993; Huse 1975). A service specialization in cardiovascular care may be developed to meet a hospital's strategic goal of providing heart and vascular care in the local community. Alfred's implementation of efficiencies (allowing the physicians to buy new equipment and the staff to receive pay increases) also illustrates change that meets the organizational mission.

6.2 THE CHANGE PROCESS: ENVISIONING AND IMPLEMENTING CHANGE

Envisioning change

The process by which decision makers picture the future of operations.

Various members of an organization participate in bringing about successful managed change. How leaders **envision change**, how managers and staff **implement the change,** and how **change recipients** respond to the change all influence the outcome. Consider the case of Alfred at the Utah health clinics.

ENVISIONING CHANGE

Implementing change

The process by which managers carry out the vision of the future of operations.

The owners of the clinics (i.e., the physicians) wanted to respond effectively to the environmental changes of reimbursement schedules and technology demands. They had directed Alfred to bring about efficient office management protocols for the three clinics. However, Mariana's comments that she did not understand why Alfred wanted to change everything indicate that the physicians and Alfred may be the only ones in the clinics who understand why the changes are needed. The physicians wanted to purchase new equipment (to respond to environmental and technological demands) and raise the salaries of the staff (to remain in accordance with the clinics' mission). Simply put, a vision motivated the change at the higher administrative levels in the clinics.

Change recipients

The staff members whose work behaviors may be affected by changes implemented.

Collins and Porras (1991) discuss the importance of creating a shared organizational vision. They present a vision framework that encompasses the firm's guiding philosophy (i.e., values, beliefs, and purpose) and a tangible image (i.e., mission and a vivid description of the outcome). The final product of the firm's vision is therefore clear and shared. Alfred's dilemma has resulted from the absence of a clear, shared vision. A critical factor of successful change is consistent, clear communication of the vision to everyone responsible for making the change happen.

IMPLEMENTING CHANGE

Alfred has a problem to address at the Utah health clinics, and it goes beyond getting Mariana "on board." Alfred is responsible for implementing the efficiency changes successfully, and he is not succeeding. None of his ideas have been implemented in the clinics. Mariana's **resistance to change** has successfully delayed Alfred's plans.

Lewin (1947) introduced the concept of resistance to change in social science. He proposed that successful change has three aspects: **unfreezing**, moving, and **refreezing**. Unfreezing refers to reducing the forces that are keeping an organization in its current state. Moving refers to implementing the change (e.g., Alfred's implementation of the new patient database). Refreezing refers to stabilizing the forces and making the newly implemented change part of the organization (Lewin 1947). Alfred is caught in the *unfreezing* stage, to use Lewin's terminology. Mariana's resistance shows that Alfred's pressure for change has not significantly altered her desire to maintain the current condition.

According to Lewin, our understanding of an employee's behavior rests upon our understanding of that person and the environment in which he operates. While change may affect the person and the work environment, the manager has more control over the environment. Thus, a manager may help bring about conditions that allow for effective change by assessing and altering the environment. Lewin introduced the term "resistance to change" as a concept that affects managers and employees (Burnes 2007). Change occurs when the driving forces for change increase and the resistance forces against change decrease. A manager may be able to create an effective change implementation plan by properly identifying the driving and restraining forces for change.

The successful implementation of change also depends on a manager's ability to reduce the resistance to change. Questions to assess change implementation include: "How did we introduce the change ideas?" "What has been the response of those affected by the change?" "What, if anything, should we do differently?" A lack of effective communication is apparent between Alfred and the office managers in the three clinics. Additionally, he has not considered the reasons for the resistance to his efficiency plan. Did he introduce his ideas well? Has he identified the driving and restraining forces for change?

Kanter, Stein, and Jick (1992) recommend three events for beginning a **change process**. The first event is providing directed, action-oriented information to all **stakeholders**. A "stakeholder" is any individual or group with a direct interest in the organization. Employees, customers, other institutions, and shareholders of a for-profit business may have a vested interest in the change. Alfred's stakeholders are the physicians, the office managers, the general office staff, and (depending on the specific change implemented)

Resistance to change
Change recipients' hesitation or refusal to comply with the vision of the future of operations and management attempts at carrying out the vision.

Unfreezing
Reducing the forces that are keeping an organization in its current state.

Refreezing
Stabilizing the forces that have brought about a newly implemented change so they become part of the organization.

Change process
The process whereby managed changed is envisioned and implemented (successfully or unsuccessfully) in an organization.

the patients. Consistent and clear communication with them would help to implement change successfully.

When Alfred met with the clinics' office managers, he informed them of changes to come. As Alfred assesses how well he introduced his ideas, he should consider Kanter, Stein, and Jick's (1992) stakeholder recommendation. He should also consider the need for staff in the vision of efficiency. Following Collins and Porras (1991), including the staff would help to create and get endorsement for a vision.

The second event Kanter, Stein, and Jick (1992) propose is building on platforms that are already in place. The office managers may be able to help perfect Alfred's general efficiency plan precisely because they have direct experience. Alfred would be reinforcing the staff's awareness of and involvement in the future direction of the clinics while potentially improving his plan. The third event is encouraging problem solving and small, incremental experimentation that departs from tradition without destroying it. Clinic managers could propose ideas for and then be a part of the change process to learn what works for the clinics and what does not. The final outcome is that the staff is involved in the change process, they are empowered by the changes, and they have participated in shaping the future of the clinics.

Arndt (1996) applied the Kanter, Stein, and Jick (1992) recommendations to a hospital social work department. She found that the process enabled the department to create a shared vision for the future and to participate in bringing about the changes. Specifically, the outcome of meetings, shared dialogue, consistent communication, and brainstorming was corporate commitment, individual empowerment, and professional growth. Unlike Alfred, Arndt (1996) was able to implement change successfully in the hospital social work department. As staff members became involved in the process, they began to own the project; thus, resistance was not an issue.

Consistent communication is important in bringing about successful change. Sharing the vision goes beyond just telling employees what changes are occurring. Lewis (2007) presents a communication model for change implementation. She concurs with the recommendation of Kanter, Stein, and Jick (1992) and supports communication that includes stakeholder recognition and input. As noted earlier, Alfred had neglected to involve Mariana and the other office managers in the process. Hence, Alfred feels Mariana's resistance to change keenly as his plans flounder. Kanter (2001) asserts that people may resist changes for reasons that make sense to them. She offers ten classic reasons why people resist change (see box).

Several of these reasons may explain Mariana's resistance to Alfred's plan. She has worked at the primary care clinic for over 20 years, and this tenure allows her a place of honor. Alfred has introduced changes without consulting her, which may cause Mariana to fear losing that place of honor. This is Kanter's (2001) number one resistance reason. In addition, she was not part of the decision-making process and may fear a loss of control (reason two), and the change plan involves performing work in a different way than it is currently being performed (reason five).

> ## (✴) KANTER'S (2001) TEN CLASSIC REASONS PEOPLE RESIST CHANGE
>
> 1. **Loss of face.** Individuals may be concerned that they will lose their place of honor and a degree of dignity.
> 2. **Loss of control.** Individuals may be concerned that they are not part of the decision-making process and are losing power.
> 3. **Excess uncertainty.** Individuals may not know what is going on or what will happen next, and they may feel unsure of what this change means.
> 4. **Surprise, surprise!** Individuals do not have advance warning and little to no chance to prepare themselves for the change.
> 5. **The "difference" effect.** Individuals may reject the change because it does not fit with the current way of doing work. The change presents unfamiliar challenges to the way work is currently performed.
> 6. **"Can I do it?"** Individuals may be concerned about their competence once the change is implemented.
> 7. **Ripple effects.** Individuals may experience changes and disruptions to their other work activities and the negative effect the change may have on these tasks.
> 8. **More work.** Individuals may resist because they do not have the time to learn new procedures or tasks, and the change may increase their workloads.
> 9. **Past resentments.** Individuals have memories of unresolved negative experiences with those involved in implementing the change. They resist the change because of their resentments toward the people involved in the process.
> 10. **Real threats.** Individuals may perceive the change to be a real threat that will result in real losses to them as the recipients of change.
>
> (Kanter 2001, 256–7) Copyright © 2001 by Harvard Business Publishing; all rights reserved. Reprinted with permission.

Beer, Eisenstat, and Spector (1990) propose a six-step model to help bring about effective change, reduce resistance, and effect Lewin's (1947) unfreezing, moving, and refreezing change aspects. The first step is to diagnose the problem and create the incentive for change. In this step, stakeholder input is used to define current conditions and to identify what change is needed. Mariana, as a clinic office manager, did not understand why Alfred wanted to change the patient database. However, if Alfred had requested her input, they could have discussed the separate protocols for patient filing in Mariana's office. Separate protocols may allow a patient to interact independently with each clinic, and one clinic may not be aware that a patient had been seen in another. A central database would ensure that all clinics are aware of all patient interactions. Given an opportunity to diagnose, Alfred and the three office managers could have diagnosed potential problems with the current patient filing system, and Alfred could have generated support for the solution of a central patient database.

Second, Beer, Eisenstat, and Spector (1990) propose the development of a shared vision. The first two steps, stakeholder participation and effective communication, are essential. Once the core team commits to a vision, change that fits with that vision can be introduced. The manager role is a factor for the third step. It is not enough to endorse a shared vision; action should follow. The manager helps foster implementation of change actions. Alfred could provide support to office managers as they implement the change. He could meet with them on a regular basis or allow for additional clerical assistance for data entry of the patient information. The fourth step is to include the staff in the decision making. Alfred could, for example, allow the office managers to try various types of database software and ask for their feedback. Fifth is the establishment of the change through formal policies and structures. The entry of patient information into the new central database ensures that this change is part of the clinic protocol. The last step is monitoring and responding to problems in the change process. The purpose of Alfred's plan was to create efficiencies. If the data entry clerks do not know how to enter the data properly, for instance, the change will not be an asset. If Mariana is still not on board, Alfred needs to know. Monitoring implementation is key to success.

RESPONDING TO RECIPIENTS OF CHANGE

The role of the recipient of change is a significant factor for successful implementation. As the recipients of change, the employees have experience with the problem that needs to be addressed. If managers can reduce resistance and build staff commitment to the change, they are more likely to experience successful outcomes.

To address the resistance, Kanter (2001) suggests staff participation. She also advocates for a shared vision and honest communication about the changes. Consistent demonstrations of the commitment to change and clearly outlined expectations help to reduce staff resistance.

Throughout the change process, the importance of the stakeholder role should be emphasized. Using Lewin's (1947) terms, stakeholder input helps to unfreeze, and their actions help to move. After refreezing, the newly implemented change becomes part of the organization.

Assessment

The act of determining the importance or value of some action, procedure, or structure.

6.3 CHANGE ASSESSMENT

An **assessment** of the change aids in refreezing. For change to be meaningful, it should add value and offer a good fit with organizational mission and vision. For Alfred, the centralized database will add value by creating efficiencies for the clinic offices. A measurement of exactly which efficiencies worked well and which did not provides insight into the change process. Furthermore, the assessment can help create a foundation for future change initiatives. Bartunek and colleagues (2006) assessed the reaction of nurses to change initiatives at their workplaces. Their findings indicated a positive response to the change; the nurses approved of the empowerment the change offered them. Their participation in the process helped bring about successful outcomes.

Evaluations of change initiatives offer a clear framework for examining what went right with the process, and what went wrong. Managers who assess the process should answer who, what, where, when, why, and how questions. Who introduced the change ideas? What was presented, and what was the stakeholder response? Where did the change occur in the organization? Why was the change needed at this time? How long did the process take? What was the timeline for implementation? How does the change fit in with organizational mission? What, if anything, should have been done differently?

Alfred has a problem. His efficiency plan is failing. To effectively address his problem, he should ask the questions of who, what, where, when, why, and how. He could reintroduce the change plan by meeting with the stakeholders (the three clinic office managers). During this meeting, he could ask for their input, their participation, and their assessment of efficiency needs at the clinics. With that meeting and with continued, consistent supportive efforts, Alfred may be able to get Mariana to build a commitment to change, giving the change a better chance to succeed.

DISCUSSION QUESTIONS

➤ Evaluate the statement that the role of the stakeholder is important for successful change implementation. Give an example from your own experience that illustrates this importance.

➤ Alfred's problem implementing his efficiency plan had to do with what he did *not* do. Assess his performance by determining the questions of who, what, when, where, why, and how he should have addressed with the staff at the WPHC when he first started his new job and then answering them.

➤ With reference to Kanter's (2001) ten classic reasons people resist change, how would you recommend a manager should introduce a new work schedule that includes weekend work for staff used to working only on weekdays?

EXERCISE 6.1 THE DIRECTOR WANTS PATIENT ERROR REDUCTION

Hank Collins is the director of the pediatrics department at St. Anthony's Catholic Hospital in Rhode Island. Annually, about 4,000 children are treated as inpatients, and over 20,000 receive outpatient care. Hank wants to implement a program to help prevent medical errors in the care of children. Specifically, he wants the staff to adopt the U.S. Department of Health and Human Services' (2002) *20 Tips to Help Prevent Medical Errors in Children* (see box). He has already posted the tips in the pediatric waiting room and at the nurses' station, and now he wants the staff to sign the postings to show they agree with the tips. Furthermore, he wants the staff to wear buttons that read, "Ask me if I have washed my hands."

---

 20 TIPS TO HELP PREVENT MEDICAL ERRORS IN CHILDREN

Be Involved in Your Child's Healthcare

1. **The single most important way you can help to prevent errors is to be an active member of your child's healthcare team.**

   That means taking part in every decision about your child's healthcare. Research shows that parents who are more involved with their child's care tend to get better results. Some specific tips, based on the latest scientific evidence about what works best, follow.

Medicines

2. **Make sure all of your child's doctors know about everything your child is taking and his or her weight. This includes prescription and over-the-counter medicines and dietary supplements such as vitamins and herbs.**

   At least once a year, bring all of your child's medicines and supplements with you to the doctor. "Brown bagging" your child's medicines can help you and your doctor talk about them and find out if there are any problems. Knowing your child's medication history and weight can help your doctor keep your child's records up to date, which can help your child get better quality care.

(✱) 20 TIPS TO HELP PREVENT MEDICAL ERRORS IN CHILDREN

3. **Make sure your child's doctor knows about any allergies and how your child reacts to medicines.**

   This can help you avoid getting a medicine that can harm your child.

4. **When your child's doctor writes you a prescription, make sure you can read it.**

   If you can't read the doctor's handwriting, your pharmacist might not be able to either. Ask the doctor to use block letters to print the name of the drug.

5. **When you pick up your child's medicine from the pharmacy, ask, "Is this the medicine that my child's doctor prescribed?"**

   A study by the Massachusetts College of Pharmacy and Allied Health Sciences found that 88 percent of medicine errors involved the wrong drug or the wrong dose.

6. **Ask for information about your child's medicines in terms you can understand—both when the medicines are prescribed and when you receive them at the hospital or pharmacy.**

   • What is the name of the medicine?

   • What is the medicine for?

   • Is the dose of this medicine appropriate for my child based on his or her weight?

   • How often is my child supposed to take it, and for how long?

   • What side effects are likely? What do I do if they occur?

   • Is this medicine safe for my child to take with other medicines or dietary supplements?

   • What food, drink, or activities should my child avoid while taking this medicine?

   • When should I see an improvement?

7. **If you have any questions about the directions on your child's medicine labels, ask.**

   Medicine labels can be hard to understand. For example, ask if "four doses daily" means taking a dose every six hours around the clock or just during regular waking hours.

   (Continued)

20 TIPS TO HELP PREVENT MEDICAL ERRORS IN CHILDREN

8. **Ask your pharmacist for the best device to measure your child's liquid medicine. Also, ask questions if you're not sure how to use the device.**

   Research shows that many people do not understand the right way to measure liquid medicines. For example, many use household teaspoons, which often do not hold a true teaspoon of liquid. Special devices, like marked oral syringes, help people to measure the right dose. Being told how to use the devices helps even more.

9. **Ask for written information about the side effects your child's medicine could cause.**

   If you know what might happen, you will be better prepared if it does—or if something unexpected happens instead. That way, you can report the problem right away and get help before it gets worse. A study found that written information about medicines can help people recognize problem side effects. If your child experiences side effects, alert the doctor and pharmacist right away.

Hospital Stays

10. **If you have a choice, choose a hospital at which many children have the procedure or surgery your child needs.**

    Research shows that patients tend to have better results when they are treated in hospitals that have a great deal of experience with their condition. Find out how many of the procedures have been performed at the hospital. While your child is in the hospital, make sure he or she is always wearing an identification bracelet.

11. **If your child is in the hospital, ask all healthcare workers who have direct contact with your child whether they have washed their hands.**

    Handwashing is an important way to prevent the spread of infections in hospitals. Yet, it is not done regularly or thoroughly enough. A study found that when patients checked whether healthcare workers washed their hands, the workers washed their hands more often and used more soap.

(✱) 20 TIPS TO HELP PREVENT MEDICAL ERRORS IN CHILDREN

12. **When your child is being discharged from the hospital, ask his or her doctor to explain the treatment plan you will use at home.**

    This includes learning about your child's medicines and finding out when he or she can get back to regular activities. Research shows that at discharge time, doctors think people understand more than they really do about what they should or should not do when they return home.

Surgery

13. **If your child is having surgery, make sure that you, your child's doctor, and the surgeon all agree and are clear on exactly what will be done.**

    Doing surgery at the wrong site (for example, operating on the left knee instead of the right) is rare—but even once is too often. The good news is that wrong-site surgery is 100 percent preventable. The American Academy of Orthopaedic Surgeons urges its members to sign their initials directly on the site to be operated on before the surgery.

Other Steps You Can Take

14. **Speak up if you have questions or concerns.**

    You have a right to question anyone who is involved with your child's care.

15. **Make sure that you know who (such as your child's pediatrician) is in charge of his or her care.**

    This is especially important if your child has many health problems or is in a hospital.

16. **Make sure that all health professionals involved in your child's care have important health information about him or her.**

    Do not assume that everyone knows everything they need to. Don't be afraid to speak up.

17. **Ask a family member or friend to be there with you and to be your advocate.**

    Choose someone who can help get things done and speak up for you if you can't.

    (Continued)

⊛ **20 TIPS TO HELP PREVENT MEDICAL ERRORS IN CHILDREN**

18. Ask why each test or procedure is being done.

It is a good idea to find out why a test or treatment is needed and how it can help. Your child could be better off without it.

19. If your child has a test, ask when the results will be available.

If you don't hear from the doctor or the lab, call to ask about the test results.

20. Learn about your child's condition and treatments by asking the doctor and nurse and by using other reliable sources.

Ask your child's doctor if his or her treatment is based on the latest scientific evidence. Treatment recommendations based on the latest scientific evidence are available from the National Guideline Clearinghouse or other websites, such as Healthfinder at www.healthfinder.gov.

He has been having trouble with one of his best employees. Anne Gordon is 55 years old and has been with the hospital for 35 years. She started out as a new graduate from the local university's LPN nursing program, and she rarely misses a day of work. She is helpful, friendly, and smart. She knows the departmental procedures (e.g., making the patients and their families feel cared for, ensuring quality in patient delivery) better than anyone, and she prides herself on the fact that many of the younger employees come to her for help. She takes particular pride in being their mentor.

However, Anne will not sign the postings and has adamantly refused to wear the button that reads, "Ask me if I have washed my hands." She is vocal about her disapproval. "How demeaning is it to be asked to wear a button on my uniform? Buttons are for political candidates to wear during political campaigns; they are not for us to wear as we take care of patients! And signing the posting would be like admitting that I had committed medical errors. No way am I going to be involved with this cockamamie idea!"

➤ What is the problem, and what is causing it?

➤ What should Hank do to gain Anne's endorsement? What recommendations do Kanter, Stein, and Jick (1992) make that might help Hank?

➤ Recommend a solution to the problem. Why do you think your solution will work?

EXERCISE 6.2   LEWIN'S FORCE FIELD

Please refer to the mission statement and strategic plan of Tenniken Medical University (TMU) as you consider your response to this exercise.

MISSION STATEMENT OF TENNIKEN MEDICAL UNIVERSITY

Tenniken Medical University (TMU) is a public institution of higher learning. Its purpose is to preserve and optimize human life in South Carolina. The university provides an environment for learning and discovery through the education of healthcare professionals and biomedical scientists, research in the health sciences, and provision of comprehensive healthcare. The university is committed to fulfilling the following responsibilities:

- To educate students to become caring, compassionate, ethical, and proficient healthcare professionals and creative biomedical scientists

- To recruit and develop dedicated, scholarly teachers who inspire their students to lifelong learning in the service of human health

- To offer educational opportunities to graduates, faculty, and staff; to other biomedical scientists and practicing health professionals; and to the public

- To seek and welcome students, scholars, and staff regardless of gender, race, age, nationality, religion, or disability, recognizing the benefits of diversity

- To conduct research in the health sciences, advancing knowledge and encouraging new responses to healthcare needs

- To provide excellence in patient care, in an environment that is respectful of others, adaptive to change, accountable for outcomes, and attentive to the needs of underserved populations

- To advance economic development by introducing new technology and fostering research links with industry and other academic institutions

- To optimize the use of all resources, including financial support from the state and revenues generated from research, clinical operations, and philanthropy

- To provide leadership to the state in efforts to promote health and prevent disease

- To serve as a state resource in health policy, education, and related matters for other institutions and the general public

TMU Strategic Plan

◆ Open and operate the first phase of our replacement hospital, continue planning for the next phase, and, in the process, develop a national leadership role in patient safety and clinical effectiveness

◆ Open and operate the Fast-Track Nursing Program, a program designed to address the nursing shortage.

◆ Integrate interprofessional education, research, and practice

◆ Implement a new IT program for the Family Practice Residency Program

◆ Continue to grow research centers of excellence, including recruiting outstanding faculty and adding new facilities with emphases in drug discovery and development, bioengineering, clinical research, and healthcare disparities

Decreased state financial support and a failed $300 million foundation campaign have led the TMU board of directors to reassess its strategic plan. The board members agree that the strategic plan is at risk, and they are debating which elements of the plan should be deleted or changed to reflect the current dismal economic climate. They agree that a change in priorities is a must; they simply cannot afford to meet all of the points noted in the plan. You are on a task force that has been charged with proposing which plan bullets should remain and which should be deleted. Any recommendations made by the task force must fit with the university's mission.

Develop a series of tables to help your task force discuss which changes should be recommended. Using Lewin's (1947) theory regarding the unfreezing, moving, and refreezing aspects of change, identify anticipated driving and restraining forces for change. For example,

TABLE 6.1

The Fast Track Nursing Program

Driving Force	Restraining Force
Effective use of existing funds to generate new funds	Administrative constraints on program development (cost control)
Response to community need for more nurses	Political backlash as other new programs are postponed (drug development)
Effecting quality patient care as student nurses work one on one with patients	

if the task force were to recommend implementation of the Fast Track Nursing Program, forces regarding successful implementation may be those listed in Table 6.1.

➤ With reference to your constructed tables, what are the most common driving forces for change you noted? Most common restraining forces identified?

➤ What is your recommended change plan to the board?

CHAPTER 7

TEAMWORK

Ben Delozier, director of the stroke recovery unit at St. John's Rehabilitation Institute, closed his office door and sighed. Most of the time, he liked his work. Helping someone to lead as normal a life as possible after a stroke was gratifying. The patients exerted great effort to recover, and they appreciated his and his staff's help in the rehabilitation process. Most of the time, he liked the professional staff members with whom he worked. St. John's staff members were divided into interdisciplinary teams that focused on the individual's therapy. A nurse, a speech pathologist, an audiologist, a physical therapist (PT), and an occupational therapist (OT) would come together to plan, implement, and evaluate the specific rehabilitation treatment for a patient. The team members, who are from about the same hierarchical level, work together to help the patient recover. "Restore the body, empower the spirit" is a philosophy to which the team members subscribe. That is, they subscribe to it most of the time.

Ben sighed again and said to himself, "Today is not one of those times." Nurse Julie Turner, audiologist Amelia Torres, and speech pathologist Martin Smith had spoken with him about the behavior of two of their interdisciplinary team members: Joseph Sarducci from PT and Vince Antoni from OT. Amelia had explained that Joseph and Vince never get along. Each one is great to work with individually.

Joseph is friendly and helpful. He was one of the first physical therapists St. John's had hired 30 years ago. He knows the rehab unit's procedures better than anyone, and is a well respected PT. He conscientiously keeps up to date with treatments and protocol, and many of the other PTs come to Joseph for consultation. Joseph says that he likes helping staff help patients "restore the body and empower the spirit."

Vince Antoni is 26 years old and graduated from the local university's OT program last year. This is his first full-time employment, and he is full of energy, full of ideas, and always ready to take on the next task. In fact, Vince sometimes gets so excited about an idea that it is difficult to get him to stop talking so others can express their opinions.

Martin had told Ben that when Joseph and Vince are working on the same team, they never get along. They argue about anything and everything. If Vince recommends a particular course of action, Joseph opposes it. And it is difficult for Joseph to get a word in, so when he does have the opportunity to talk, he ends up shouting at Vince. Their interaction is not helping them help the patient.

Amelia added, "When we tell them to stop fighting and get back to discussing the patient, they pout and refuse to participate."

Julie concluded by adding, "We just end up frustrated with the time wasted. They are both so busy trying to lead the team and telling everyone else what to do that we don't get to accomplish as much as we could."

After studying this chapter, you will be able to

➤ recognize the role of interdisciplinary teams in healthcare organizations,

➤ appreciate the importance of effective teams for patients and staff members,

➤ identify characteristics of effective teams, and

➤ understand the concept of groupthink.

7.1 HEALTHCARE TEAMS

The use of teams is standard practice in healthcare organizations. Dedicated clinical teams for patient care and management teams designed to develop and implement a healthcare organization's strategy, rules, and protocol exist to improve healthcare and the delivery of healthcare services.

Heinemann (2002) discusses the history of team development in the U.S. healthcare system. In the 1900s, physicians initiated the use of teams as a strategy for communicating about the patient. By the 1930s, nurses officially supported the team approach to coordinating patient care. Interdisciplinary healthcare professionals continued to endorse the use of teams in clinical practice, and by the end of the twentieth century, The Joint Commission had mandated that patient care plans document interdisciplinary input.

Collaboration and cooperation by professional members of a healthcare team have resulted in improvements in patient care. Lemieux-Charles and McGuire (2006) conducted a literature review of studies that assessed the effects of **interdisciplinary teams** on clinical outcomes. Overall, they found a positive relationship between the presence of teams and patient outcomes (see, for example, Cohen et al. 2002 and Caplan et al. 2004).

Interdisciplinary healthcare teams have employed business models such as Total Quality Improvement (TQI), Six Sigma, and Toyota Production System to improve delivery.

Interdisciplinary team
A group of people who represent different disciplines working together to accomplish a common goal.

Virtua (a four-hospital system serving southern New Jersey and Philadelphia) reduced length of stay for congestive heart failure (CHF) patients by adopting Six Sigma (Ettinger 2001). The interdisciplinary team was able to identify problems that led to increased stay and to provide best-practice solutions. CHF patients tend to be geriatric patients, and exposure to unfamiliar surroundings and the increased germ environment of a healthcare facility may introduce unnecessary negative outcomes for them.

The team identified four factors that affected lengths of stay: family expectations and education regarding CHF, nursing protocol for patient care, specific care procedures, and post-hospital care instruction. The outcome of this team approach was a reduction in patient stay from 6.2 days to 4.6 days, which benefited the geriatric patients. This outcome was also beneficial to Virtua, because it implemented efficiency-producing methods. The overall result is that effective teamwork yielded benefits to the patient and to the healthcare organization.

Research regarding the team approach supports beneficial outcomes not only for patients, but also for staff. Collaboration and cooperation of healthcare team members are positively associated with job satisfaction, and recruitment and retention are influenced by the organizational environment. If upper management supports team efforts, if team leaders are positive regarding the team, if communication is clear regarding the team's goals, and if communication among members supports the charge's importance to organizational success, positive outcomes are more likely (see, for example, Anderson 1993; Weisman et al. 1993; Barczak 1996; Borrill et al. 2000; Amos, Hu, and Herrick 2005).

The problem confronting Ben Delozier, director of the stroke recovery unit, is a team that lacks collaboration and cooperation. Ben has two concerns to address: the conflict between Joseph and Vince that may affect commitment by other team members and, more importantly, the conflict's potential interference with patient care. Ben knows that the conflict is a barrier to effective team performance, and he has several options for addressing this problem.

First, he may make certain that Joseph and Vince are not on the same interdisciplinary team. Second, he may talk with them separately to ascertain why the conflict exists and to develop a plan to address their concerns effectively. Third, he may choose not get involved and to let the team address the conflict. Ben rejects the first option, because St. John's Rehabilitation Institute is about patient care. The staff needs to learn how to behave in a professional manner to help patients. At the same time, however, Ben knows that the context in which the team operates needs to be addressed to prevent this problem from happening again. He needs to rally the team and help establish a framework for effective team construction and maintenance. Ignoring the problem is not a viable option. He decides to meet with Joseph and Vince and work on a plan of corrective action.

7.2 CHARACTERISTICS OF EFFECTIVE TEAMS

Hellriegel and Slocum (2003) developed a self-assessment tool to determine team effectiveness. The team members answer the following questions:

1. Do the members know why the team exists?

2. Do the members have a procedure for making decisions?

3. Do the members communicate freely among themselves?

4. Do the members help each other?

5. Do the members deal with conflict among themselves?

6. Do the members identify and address ways to improve the team's functioning?

If Julie, Martin, Amelia, Joseph, and Vince completed the self-assessment, their team might score poorly. While the team members understand why the team exists, evidence indicates that they do not communicate freely among themselves. Vince and Joseph are not helping one another; Joseph dismisses Vince's ideas, and Vince resists allowing others to speak. Neither are they dealing with conflict among themselves; Julie, Amelia, and Martin have turned to Ben (their supervisor) for help.

The Academic Health Center Task Force on Interdisciplinary Health Team Development (1996) list ten competencies team members should strive to accomplish. These competencies form a basis for team self-assessment.

1. Do the members focus on the patient as their first priority?

2. Do the members have established common goals regarding patient outcomes?

3. Do the members understand the roles of other team members who represent different professions?

4. Do the members have confidence in the abilities of other team members?

5. Are the members flexible in their roles to accommodate team goals?

6. Do the members share group norms and expectations?

7. Do the members deal with conflict among themselves?

8. Do the members communicate freely among themselves?

9. Do the members share responsibility for actions made by the team?

10. Do the members evaluate themselves and their team performance?

Applying the assessments of Hellriegel and Slocum (2003) and the Academic Health Center Task Force (1996) to the interdisciplinary team of Julie, Martin, Amelia, Joseph, and Vince suggests that this team is not as effective as it could be. Their uncooperative behavior has resulted in the team's accomplishing less than it could. Their team lacks the needed communication and conflict-management skills to address the problems that have occurred. Hence, three of its five members have turned to Ben for help.

7.3 STRATEGIES FOR DEVELOPING TEAM EFFECTIVENESS

Team effectiveness depends on how well the members work together. Tuckman (1965) and Tuckman and Jensen (1977) propose that individuals move through stages of team development and behavior. The stages are forming, storming, norming, performing, and adjourning. The **forming** stage is an orientation phase in which members are given their charge or purpose for the team. During this stage, team members learn about one another's personalities. The **storming** stage is characterized by conflict and emotional issues that may inhibit a team's progress toward performing the task with which it was charged. Team members learn to work effectively (or not) with one another, given their personalities.

The St. John's Rehab team is stuck in this storming stage. Joseph and Vince have allowed their conflict to overshadow work efforts, and the other team members are frustrated by the time that has been wasted. The ultimate concern is that Joseph and Vince are more focused on their conflict than they are on developing, implementing, and evaluating the patient's rehabilitation care plan. If this team is able to move forward, it will experience the **norming** stage that Tuckman (1965) proposed. In this stage, team members agree upon working styles and make compromises. Conflict is reduced as the team unifies. The energy that had been directed toward the conflict is now devoted to the charge of patient care. The team then enters the fourth stage, **performing**, and they work productively together. The final stage is **adjourning**, during which the team goes over its successes and individuals disengage from the team. As the patient is discharged from the rehabilitation unit, the team regroups to focus on a new task or a new team is created, and the process begins again.

Managers can establish an organizational context that is conducive to team success. They communicate the team's charge clearly; they set the stage for a positive and supportive environment; and they focus on the team's goal. Staff members expect managers to take the lead to establish a positive work environment (Harmon, Brallier, and Brown 2002). During the forming stage of the rehab team, Ben could have met with the members and reviewed the team's purpose, discussed the patient load for the team, and endorsed a positive work environment where team members treat one another with respect, listen to one another's ideas, and allow one another to contribute. However, the team is stuck in the storming stage, and Ben needs to decide how best to deal with the problem.

As mentioned earlier, Ben could ignore the problem, but this action would only encourage the team members who approached Ben to conclude a lack of support for them or for the team's goals. He might encourage the three team members to talk with Joseph and Vince and have the team solve the problem itself. However, Amelia has tried that without

Forming
The first stage of teamwork, during which members are given their charge or the purpose of the team.

Storming
The second stage of teamwork, during which team members learn about one another. This stage is characterized by conflict and emotional issues that may inhibit a team's progress.

Norming
The third stage of teamwork, during which team members agree upon working styles, conflict is reduced, and group cohesiveness emerges.

Performing
The fourth stage of teamwork, during which team members are engaged in the work and purpose of the team.

Adjourning
The final stage of teamwork, during which team members review outcomes and successes and individuals disengage from the team.

success. So Ben opts to meet with Joseph and Vince separately and develop a plan of correction. He also should meet with the team as a whole to create a supportive environment as it resolves its storming experiences.

As the team regroups, leadership style may also be addressed. Leadership in teams may be authoritarian, laissez-faire, or democratic. Joseph and Vince have been vying for **authoritarian** rule, but the resulting conflict suggests that authoritarian leadership may not be the best style for the team. **Laissez-faire** (hands-off) leadership may not be best either, as team members need to bring in their expertise from their different disciplines and discuss patient care specifics. At times, different team members will need to take the lead. **Democratic** (shared) leadership among the five team members may be more appropriate than Joseph and Vince vying for authoritarian rule, because the team members are from about the same hierarchical level and pool their expertise to help the patient "restore the body and empower the spirit." Research indicates that teams that experience shared leadership tend to perform better than teams with an authoritarian leader (Solansky 2008).

Ben's challenge is to figure out the best way to ensure that Joseph and Vince are fulfilling their roles as team members. Fisher, Ury, and Patton (1991) offer advice on principled negotiation with people who are in conflict with one another. First, they advocate that the problem be defined and the options outlined. Ben has accomplished this necessary step. Second, they recommend that the people be separated from the issues and that each one should try to understand the other's position. If Ben meets with Joseph and Vince, he can ask Joseph why he ignores Vince's ideas. Joseph may respond that Vince is very new to the profession and could learn more if he took time to listen. Vince may then offer his opinion that Joseph has been there more than 30 years and is a "know-it-all." As the supervisor, Ben then can direct Joseph and Vince to propose what they think might work for both parties so that the team functions better. Fisher, Ury, and Patton (1991) suggest that the more the conflicting parties are involved in the negotiation process, the more likely they are to support any initiative that addresses the problem. Ben's involvement of Joseph and Vince in the process is more likely to result in a successful outcome. As they brainstorm possible solutions, they are focusing on the ultimate goal of a healthcare team—working together on a common goal.

Additionally, Fisher, Ury, and Patton (1991) stress that each team member should allow other team members to express their emotions and listen actively to improve communication. Active listening is discussed in Chapter 6; however, the basic principles of active listening are that the receiver of the message should pay attention to the sender (speaker) and focus on the message. The receiver may summarize the message to ensure that it was being delivered clearly and correctly. Last, the speaker and receiver should respect one another throughout the process. If one party is unwilling to engage in this principled negotiation process, the other parties should keep returning the conversation to the problem at hand. This helps to keep the attention focused on solving the problem, which would allow for the team to move on to the performing stage, the ultimate goal of Ben's meeting with Joseph and Vince.

7.4 A WORD ABOUT GROUPTHINK

While the research indicates that cohesive team efforts benefit patients and staff, evidence also suggests that mistakes may occur precisely because a team is especially cohesive. Janus (1972, 1982) proposed the term "**groupthink**" to illustrate this process. Groups whose members are well-informed and intelligent but who also define themselves and their work as morally superior, are isolated from outside ideas and practices, are in a stressful work environment, possess illusions of invulnerability, and experience strong in-group cohesiveness may make decisions that are not in the best interest of patient care (Janus 1972, 1982).

One would expect healthcare teams that are in the performing stage to be generally cohesive, and one would expect that healthcare team members are extremely busy and are working under a time constraint. Healthcare professionals may spend less time outside of the healthcare arena because of the profession's work demands and, as a result, they may become isolated and even more cohesive with other team members. Healthcare is a stressful occupation, and the team may be pressured to contain costs. These factors allow for groupthink and can cause a good team to make poor decisions.

Heinemann and colleagues (1994) applied Janus's groupthink theory to the geriatric healthcare environment. They present the case of an older couple in which the wife is the primary caregiver. The husband becomes paralyzed from the neck down and the wife continues the primary caretaking responsibilities more than 18 months. Two members of the healthcare team are extremely domineering; the rest of the team is busy, under stress, and focused on cost containment for the hospital.

Communication among team members is left to the two most vocal members. Other member input is nil. Team members who exhibit a morally superior stance look down upon nursing home care, and they feel this opinion is justified by the husband's preference not to go to a nursing home.

After a year and a half, the wife is exhausted. She cannot continue to deliver the care her husband needs. When she expresses concern regarding her abilities, the team members do not listen to her, and options such as respite care or nursing home care are never introduced as viable options. The result is that the wife threatens to abandon the caregiving role. Thus, while the team members felt that the wife's caring for the husband was best for the patient, their inability to listen to her and examine other options resulted in the team's failure. The wife's leaving was certainly not in the patient's best interest.

Healthcare delivery team members need to be conscious of the potential for groupthink. They should avoid assuming the morally superior stance—because other healthcare options may fit a patient's needs well. They should also avoid isolation from other healthcare practices and protocol. A commitment to sponsor outside speakers may help a healthcare organization decrease the isolation factor. Furthermore, each team member should be allowed to be a critical evaluator. Open communication, respect for team member participation, and regularly scheduled evaluation of team behavior and performance may help prevent groupthink.

Groupthink
Conformity to group values and ethics that can lead to negative outcomes.

7.5 BEST PRACTICES GUIDELINES FOR TEAM FORMATION

Healthcare managers who rely upon team output need professional staff members who understand why the team was formed; who allow for respectful, open communication among team members; who share leadership; who deal with conflict effectively; and who evaluate team performance on a regular basis (Hellriegel and Slocum 2003; Couzins and Beagrie 2004). Healthcare managers may help by clearly defining the team goals. The team then should adhere to the following best practices:

1. Determine the best way to attain goals (what protocol may help the patient improve).

2. Agree on team norms (how team members will collaborate and communicate with one another).

3. Advocate shared leadership for interdisciplinary teams.

4. Assign specific team member functions (e.g., one member may schedule meetings, and another member may make certain that documentation for the patient is complete).

5. Hold regularly scheduled meetings.

6. Handle conflict with team members directly, but seek assistance from the supervisor if internal mechanisms do not work.

7. Evaluate team performance on a regular basis, addressing the team's strengths and weaknesses.

Healthcare managers provide a positive environment, intervene as necessary to help solve problems, and evaluate team performance. As a result, the team members are supported so they may work to "restore the body and empower the spirit."

DISCUSSION QUESTIONS

➤ Teams are currently the norm in hospital settings. Why do you think this is so? How does a team approach benefit healthcare delivery?

➤ Think of a team you have been a part of (e.g., a sports team or musical group). With reference to Hellriegel and Slocum (2003) and the Academic Health Center Task Force (1996) assessment plan, evaluate your team. Was it successful, according to the assessment criteria? Why or why not?

➤ When is an authoritarian leadership style more effective for teams? A democratic style of leadership? A laissez-faire style? Which do you think is more appropriate for teams dedicated to healthcare delivery? Why?

EXERCISE 7.1   GROUPTHINK AND THE BOARD OF GOVERNORS

The physicians of Beachside Medical Group had spent more than five years combining seven local practices into a single, multispecialty group practice. The goal of this merger was to bring the best, most respected practices together to create efficiencies in clinic management. It also gave the doctors a more powerful bargaining position in negotiations with insurance companies on policies and payment structures. The group had also introduced a radiology center, which would not have been possible if the practices had remained separate. Beachside Medical Group was now made up of 20 physicians, five physician assistants, ten nurses, three radiology technologists, one clinic manager, and six general staff and office assistants.

The governing board of Beachside Medical Group would make decisions about third-party contract negotiations, resource allocations, and strategy for the group's future. The six board members were all physicians. They noted that the representation was skewed toward a physician perspective, but they were satisfied that they would represent all interests and take their commitment to the group seriously. After all, they were the ones who were in charge and had volunteered to serve on the board.

The board met on a monthly basis for the first year to deal with all of the new clinic's business activities. Sometimes they asked Leslie Duncan, the clinic manager, to attend; sometimes they did not include Leslie. They made resolutions and passed them without input from the other physicians in the practice or from the clinic staff. After all, they knew best. They were the doctors who had volunteered. The result was that the board often met without notifying other clinic physicians and staff. Closed-door meetings became the norm.

Some of the new rules being passed frustrated Leslie. "The board is creating a series of problems for the staff. They are creating a mess, and I do not know how much longer I can continue to clean up after them." The previous month, the board had mandated a change in working schedules for the office staff. They had changed eight-hour days to ten-hour days without consulting Leslie or the staff members who would be affected by the change. This change in working hours meant that those staff members with children needed to change their childcare arrangements to accommodate the board's rules, and all staff members needed to change their day-to-day routines.

Two office assistants quit out of frustration, and Leslie was left to find qualified assistants to fill the positions quickly. She had just succeeded when the board issued two new mandates. The first was that all promised annual pay raises for staff would be postponed until the following quarter because profits had been lower than expected. The second was that all office personnel except for the physicians would punch a time clock so their hours could be documented. The staff members who had not quit after the schedule changes had stayed primarily because they were proud of their contributions to the multispecialty practice. Leslie questioned the decision not to follow through on a promised pay raise because of lower than expected profits while at the same time incurring an expense to add a monitoring system (the time clock). Leslie asked the board if she could talk about the new policy with them, and they agreed to meet with her today.

➤ What do you think Leslie should say to the board members when she meets with them?

➤ With reference to the concept of groupthink, how do you think the board made the decisions Leslie is questioning?

➤ What will the repercussions be if the board members go unchecked? What do you think will happen to staff–physician relations?

EXERCISE 7.2   NEW TEAM FORMATION AND THE REDUCTION OF PATIENT ERRORS

Grace Hunter, the vice president for strategic management, listened to Oli Bordeux, the CEO. They were discussing a new strategic initiative to eliminate patient errors. In the past five years, the 336-bed hospital they worked for had reported nine adverse patient errors that had resulted in death or a permanent vegetative state. Grace knew that they did not compare favorably with other hospitals in their area. Virginia Hope, 50 miles away and licensed for 1,400 beds, had reported four incidents and no deaths in the past five years. Swan Valley Medical Center, 80 miles away and licensed for 450 beds, had reported five incidents and three deaths in same time period.

Oli said to Grace, "I need you to form a team to deal with this. And, Grace, I need this team to find us some answers. Put together a team that can underscore the need for every staff member to step up. We need to identify potential problems before they become errors that affect our patients and their families."

Grace promised Oli that she would do what he had asked. As she left Oli's office, she said to herself, "I just need to get the right people to commit to making a difference, and then to get them to make the difference. Not an easy task."

➤ What advice would you offer Grace regarding who should be on this team? What advice would you offer regarding the team's forming phase?
➤ How should the team evaluate its own performance?
➤ How should Grace evaluate the team's performance?

PART III

INTERPERSONAL TECHNIQUES FOR MANAGERS

CHAPTER 8

COMMUNICATION

AN ABSENT-MINDED PROFESSOR

Susan Morrison excitedly approached Dr. Hans Lackenski's office. She had scheduled this appointment with her human resources in healthcare professor two weeks earlier. Susan was working toward a BS in healthcare administration, and she had a great idea for her senior paper. Each student was to present an idea to a professor and ask that professor to serve as the advisor for the paper. Susan enjoyed studying healthcare administration. Her GPA was 3.75 on a 4.0 scale, and she had taken Dr. Lackenski's course the previous semester.

Susan was interested in working in human resources, particularly on recruitment and retention issues for healthcare professionals. In Dr. Lackenski's HR class, Susan had learned that hospitals, nursing homes, and clinics were engaging in nontraditional methods to recruit nurses. She had an associate's degree in nursing and had earned her RN degree five years earlier. She had been working at the university hospital ever since, and she had maintained her work schedule even after she returned to school to earn her BS. She had first-hand experience with the nursing shortage. It was not uncommon for her to be called back to the hospital to work extra shifts. She also knew that her RN experience would add value to her future work as a hospital administrator. She had been researching the nursing shortage in the United States and wanted to ask Dr. Lackenski to serve as her advisor and to guide her with his expertise on recruitment and retention issues.

The department secretary ushered Susan into Dr. Lackensi's office. Dr. Lackenski was sitting at his desk, looking at the computer screen. He waved for Susan to sit down and said—without moving his eyes from the computer screen—"What can I do for you?"

Susan began to talk about her research efforts. "Dr. Lackenski, I wanted to ask you what you thought about the current U.S. hospital recruitment practice of hiring nurses from other countries, such as Canada, English-speaking Caribbean and African countries, Great Britain, India, and the Philippines. Don't you think that this is really a short-term solution to the nursing shortage?" Susan leaned forward in her chair and awaited Dr. Lackenski's response.

Dr. Lackenski hit a few keys on his computer and shifted in his chair. He stopped typing for a moment and looked at his wristwatch. "Yes, there is a nursing shortage." He stood up and walked over to a file cabinet. On top of the cabinet was a tray labeled "In Box." He selected a few of the letters from the box and proceeded to open them.

Susan repeated her interest in learning his opinion on the recruiting practice. The professor kept his eyes focused on his mail. He did not appear to be interested in the topic or in her as a student at that moment. Susan asked, "Is this a bad time for you? Should I reschedule our appointment?" Dr. Lackenski looked at Susan. "Can you hold on for a minute?" He then left his office to give the letter he had been reading to the secretary.

Susan mumbled, "I see you are busy at the moment. Thank you for your time, Dr. Lackenski." She followed Dr. Lackenski out of the office. Nonplussed, she walked down the hall wondering if her professor was as smart as she had thought. What was she going to do about her senior paper?

LEARNING OBJECTIVES

After studying this chapter, you will be able to

➤ illustrate the importance of effective verbal and nonverbal communication,

➤ identify the components of communication (sender, receiver, and message),

➤ recognize the value of attentive listening, and

➤ present a case for the importance of writing well.

8.1 COMMUNICATION MATTERS

Professor-student collaboration creates an educational exchange of value that benefits the students, the professors, and the university learning community. A collaborative relationship depends on **effective communication**. In the case study, Dr. Lackenski does not appear to be engaged in this collaboration, leaving Susan to ponder what to do about her paper. However, the professor and the student may gain from effective communication and meaningful discussion. Unfortunately, this did not happen for Susan and Dr. Lackenski.

    Communication is a process whereby information is conveyed between a **sender** and a **receiver**. We know that when we communicate with our family, friends, and colleagues, the information is not always understood the way we intended. Consider the game of Gossip. One person whispers a phrase to another person; that person whispers the information to the next person, and so on. By the time the last person receives the message, it may have changed considerably.

    A recent healthcare HR class of 45 students played Gossip as a classroom exercise. They started with the following communication: "The final exam will be held on Tuesday from 1:00 p.m. to 4:00 p.m. It will have four essay questions; the student will select three of them to answer. There are also 75 multiple choice and true/false questions." When the forty-fifth student received the information, he announced the following to the class: "The exam is on Thursday from 2:00 p.m. to 4:00 p.m. It has 3 essay questions and 75 multiple

Effective communication
Communication in which the receiver receives and understands the message as the sender intended it.

Sender
The producer of a message.

Receiver
One who is given the message produced by the sender.

choice questions. No true/false questions." If this were the way the professor had communicated final exam information, many of the students would have had a stressful end to the semester. As the game of Gossip illustrates, effective communication matters.

Shannon and Weaver (1949) developed a communication model to address Bell Telephone's needs for efficient telephone cables and radio waves. Shannon and Weaver were engineers; nonetheless, their communication model became the basis for human communication research. The information source (the sender) produces the message. The transmitter (nonverbal and verbal communication) translates the message into signals. The channel refers to adaptation of voice signals to be sent over telephone cables. The channel is influenced by noise sources (any interference with the message). Shannon and Weaver (1949) were referring to phone-line static; human communication research considers any distraction that may interfere with the message to be a noise source. The receiver receives the information and decodes the message that is sent. In human communication research, the destination and the receiver are the same.

The Shannon and Weaver (1949) communication model has been simplified and adapted for human communication research (see Figure 8.1). Parsons's (2001, 13) model stresses the role of communication to inform and to persuade. Parsons states,

> In the context of your job as a healthcare manager, one of the most important reasons to consider the quality of your communication is because the relationships that you have with other individuals—and that your organization has with other groups and organizations—often originate directly from the quality of the communication that has flowed between you and others.

In the case study, Susan attempted to communicate with Dr. Lackenski about a topic for her senior paper. But was her communication clear? She neglected to explain her reason for being there, even though her nonverbal communication supported her interest in the meeting. Dr. Lackenski's **feedback** seemed to indicate disinterest. Whether he was disinterested in Susan's

Feedback
Critical assessment of information or action.

FIGURE 8.1
Communication Model for Healthcare Managers

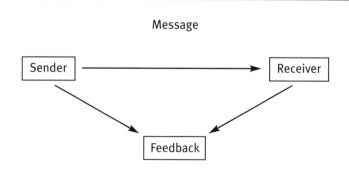

SOURCE: Adapted from Parsons (2001).

topic or in her senior paper is unclear. What is clear is that his nonverbal communication effectively told Susan that he was not listening to her and thus was not interested in the meeting. His attention to his computer screen and his mail represents the noise that may interfere with effective communication, as Shannon and Weaver (1949) indicate; this same activity represents the feedback factor illustrated in Parsons's (2001) model. The end result is that the noise and feedback Dr. Lackenski sent to Susan affected their relationship as professor and student. Susan probably will go to another professor who is willing to *listen* to her ideas, and her opinion of Dr. Lackenski will have suffered from their exchange.

8.2 ACTIVE LISTENING

A key component of communication is the receiver's ability to accurately hear what the sender is saying. This depends on whether the receiver is practicing **active listening**. According to Durutta (2006), active listening is essential for managers. The manager (sender) should check with the receiver to make certain that the message is accurately received. One method is to summarize the information and ask if this summary is accurate. Furthermore, the manager needs to allow the receiver to respond. Both parties—sender and receiver—should be willing to listen.

There are costs for parties who do not listen, in terms lost information and damaged relationships. Clark (1999), a professor at Xavier University, asked management students to recall a time when someone was actively listening to them. Students noted that they had perceived the other person was actively listening through **nonverbal** (e.g., eye contact, nodding) and **verbal cues** (e.g., repeating the information back to the speaker, asking relevant questions). They reported that they liked speaking to active listeners. The interaction indicated respect and conveyed that the receiver thought the speaker was intelligent. Further, they held the active listener in high esteem.

The opposite was found regarding student perceptions of inattentive listeners like Dr. Lackenski. They knew they were not with an active listener because of nonverbal (e.g., walking away) and verbal cues (e.g., irrelevant interruptions). The inattention caused the students anxiety, and they attributed negative qualities (e.g., arrogance and condescension) to inactive listeners.

Greenleaf (1977) proposes that learning to listen helps a manager become a servant leader, one who serves first and aspires to lead. Through active listening, this servant leader not only receives insights for effective management, but also builds strengths in those with whom she is speaking. He recommends that managers ask themselves, "Am I really listening?" when engaged in conversation. Perhaps if Dr. Lackenski had asked that question, his meeting with Susan would have been different.

Suggestions for improving listening skills include the following:

1. Stop talking. Allow the sender and receiver to speak.

2. Focus on the speaker. Use nonverbal and verbal cues to indicate your interest in what the speaker is saying.

Active listening

The process of paying close attention to a message so that it is sent and received accurately.

Nonverbal cues

In communication theory, the behaviors of persons who are interacting with one another. Body language, posture, and facial expressions may elaborate the message that is being sent or received.

Verbal cues

In communication theory, the tone and manner of the message sent and received.

3. Respect the other person. Take time to listen.

4. Be careful with interpretations. Avoid making assumptions. Ask questions to clarify what the speaker is saying.

5. Avoid distracting actions, such as looking at mail or shuffling papers. These behaviors give the impression that the receiver is not interested.

6. Do not interrupt. Let the speaker finish the thought before responding.

7. Do not talk while the other is talking. One cannot listen while speaking.

The challenge of an effective communication process is understanding how to speak and listen well.

Dye and Garman (2006) propose that effective listening skills are a critical competency for healthcare executives. Healthcare managers who listen well are not merely waiting for their turn to speak in the conversation. Rather, they are engaged in

1. maintaining a calm, easy-to-approach demeanor;

2. practicing patience with the speaker;

3. showing a willingness to listen;

4. developing an understanding of the speaker and recognizing the meaning of their messages;

5. making the effort needed to build rapport; and

6. presenting warmth and graciousness (70).

Active listening may not always create effective rapport or provide the answer to a problem, but adopting active listening skills will certainly secure an advantage.

Dr. Lackenski only engaged in the first two of Dye and Garman's (2006) recommendations: He was calm and patient. However, he did not listen as though he meant it. He may have been interested in directing Susan's paper on the nursing shortage, but his lack of attention negated his opportunity to do so. Effective communication requires that the sender send a clear message to the receiver and receive clear feedback from the receiver. In an ideal situation, Dr. Lackenski would have listened closely, acknowledged his understanding of the messages Susan presented to him, and sent his own messages back clearly. If he was unable to attend to the conversation for some reason, he should have rescheduled the meeting. One of a manager's responsibilities is to assess and respond to a situation as appropriately as one can. If Dr. Lackenski had rescheduled and listened attentively to Susan's next attempt to discuss her paper, the outcome could have been better.

8.3 INTERNAL AND EXTERNAL COMMUNICATIONS

Managers communicate with a variety of groups and individuals. Within the organization, managers interact with their bosses, their colleagues, and their staff. Staff expect their managers to share pertinent organizational information and to explain how that information will affect their work efforts (Whitworth 2006). Communication flows may be downward (e.g., CEO to department head), upward (e.g., nurse to nurse manager), or lateral (e.g., radiology technologist discussing work matters with another radiology technologist). **Downward communication** is primarily informational and initiated by the superior in the organization. Such communications are not solely face-to-face interaction. An e-mail that explains a clinic's vacation policy guidelines is an example of this form. **Upward communications** primarily let managers know about staff issues. Katz (1974) suggests that face-to-face communication in the form of open meetings to discuss employees' concerns, open-door policies, and walking the halls help create effective forums for this type of communication.

   Lateral communication is usually focused on work processes. How the work may be made more efficient, more customer friendly, and more patient centered is an example of a communication topic among colleagues with the same status. Two radiology technologists debating the most efficient way to take a number of portable X-rays exemplifies lateral communication. When lateral communication pertains to work functions, it may lead to positive outcomes in workload and efficiencies. However, lateral communication may also have negative consequences. Staff members who manipulate information for their own advantage or who offer misinformation may cause conflicts among other staff members. Managers should identify and deal with these conflicts to address such negative outcomes. (See Chapter 11 for more discussion of conflict resolution.)

   Such interpersonal skills are also important for healthcare managers in an external setting, such as with media interaction. Health and healthcare are newsworthy, and the manager as liaison helps the public understand the healthcare issues that are under scrutiny. Plain language and honesty are keys to success. Successful communication efforts with the media build relationships.

   Consider, for example, managers in not-for-profit hospitals who are trying to communicate budget expenses for community benefits. A community benefit is a program developed by a not-for-profit hospital to serve and to increase health awareness in the community around it. Not-for-profit hospitals receive tax-exempt status because of their community benefit efforts. A hospital must communicate clear community benefit messages to maintain this tax-exempt status. Clear community benefit messages are also central to a hospital's ability to inform community members about its efforts on their behalf. Common community benefit programs include community health education, screenings, immunizations, and education of healthcare professionals. Hospitals may also donate free bicycle helmets or offer childbirth classes. This allows the hospital to become familiar with the community and to show the benefits they provide (Buchmueller and Feldstein 1996). Regular, clear,

Downward communication
Communication that is primarily informational and initiated by the superior in the organization.

Upward communication
Communication that allows supervisors to know about staff members' concerns, issues, or recommendations.

Lateral communication
Communication between staff members of the same status.

consistent, honest communication with media representatives about community benefit efforts allow for future communication efforts between the hospital and the public via media
representatives.

8.4 WRITTEN COMMUNICATION

Letters, memos, reports, and PowerPoint presentations are central to the healthcare
business. Effective written communication is important, as it is relatively permanent,
retrievable, and, at times, legally binding. Parsons (2001) offers direct writing advice to
healthcare managers. Accuracy, truthfulness, and purposefulness convey the facts and
provide the reader with truthful and useful information. Clear, organized, complete, and
appropriately targeted writing helps the reader understand the information.

Effective communication includes accepting the responsibility to hone one's
writing skills. Managers should be able to write well, and they can improve via proper
training. This idea is as appropriate today as it was when it was written for the *Harvard
Business Review* in the 1950s. Gratto Liebler and McConnell (2008) offer a series of
guidelines to help managers improve their writing skills. As Parsons (2001) does, they
stress the importance of targeted writing. Managers should know who the reader is and
how well the reader knows the subject matter. This helps the manager select a writing
style and determine which information to include. If the audience is the manager's
primary team, an informal style may be appropriate. The amount of background and
detail material will vary according to the audience. The general community's need to
know will differ from an internal department's need to know, for example. Gratto
Liebler and McConnell (2008) encourage managers to use only the words necessary to
make the point—to be clear and concise. Last, to develop writing skills, they encourage
managers to edit, rewrite, and review.

DISCUSSION QUESTIONS

➤ Give some examples of verbal and nonverbal cues. How do they help or hinder effective
communication?

➤ How might managers use lateral communication to their benefit?

➤ Why do you think people tend not to engage in active listening?

EXERCISE 8.1   EFFECTIVE COMMUNICATION AND LOUIS'S CHALLENGE

Rena Lars is the supervisor for PT/OT at the University Medical Center. She and Louis Hernandez, the supervisor for radiology technology, walked down the corridor to the monthly supervisors' meeting. As they proceeded down the hallway, Louis saw Dalton Bradford, a radiology tech. Dalton had just completed his BS in radiographic sciences and had been working at the medical center for a little more than two weeks. Louis asked Rena to wait for a moment, and he headed over to where Dalton was standing.

"Dalton," Louis called out, "Have you finished taking the portable X-rays for the three inpatients?"

Dalton replied that he was still working on them and would be finished in an hour or so. He said, "I'm waiting for Mr. Dillon to get out of —"

Louis interrupted Dalton, yelling, "I don't want to hear your excuses. Just get those X-rays taken."

Louis returned to Rena, who looked alarmed. "Really, Louis," Rena said. "I don't think you needed to yell at him. You didn't hear his reason for not being finished."

Louis explained to Rena, "I'm frustrated by the techs' attitudes. You think I'm critical of them? You think I raise my voice? Well, of course I'm critical. Of course I'm loud. I have to be—they don't listen to me otherwise. If you asked them about the department, they would say that things are just fine, and Rena, they fight every change I try to implement. They have no appreciation for the importance of keeping on schedule."

If Louis was critical of his staff, it was mutual. They universally disliked him. Rena knew that the radiology techs and Louis had problems. Rad techs had been known to say: "He's totally out of touch. I just shut down and stop listening when he yells and screams at us."

One added, "I'd been working here for 12 years when he started. This was a good place to work. Not anymore. I'm constantly in fear of being chewed out. I feel stressed all the time, even at home. My wife is asking me to start looking for a job at St. Regis Medical, and I think I am going to do so."

When Louis had been hired at the medical center a year before, he was given the charge to get the radiology techs to work more. They had a reputation for slacking off and taking X-rays when they wanted to rather than as quickly as possible. High on Louis's list of goals was increasing the number of patients seen and decreasing the time spent with each one, while maintaining quality of care.

Rena asked Louis, "Do you think you have problems with the staff?"

Louis replied, "Oh, yes, I do. We just cannot communicate. Rena, you seem to get along with your people. Any advice for me?"

➤ Identify the problem in this exercise.

➤ If you were Rena, what would you suggest that Louis do?

EXERCISE 8.2   A MATTER OF DEGREE

Alaska Sound Family Clinic operates with two physicians, two nurses, one clinic manager, and three office assistants. Everyone knows everyone else; everyone is friends with everyone else. The office serves families in rural Alaska, and doctors and nurses treat patients in the clinic or fly to rural sites to provide annual checkups and follow-up care to patients who cannot travel to the clinic. The two physicians have earned MD degrees, and both are held in high regard by the communities they serve. Their diplomas are framed and hang on the wall in the clinic waiting room.

The clinic's two nurses—Sarah, hired six years ago, and Christy, hired almost a year ago—had reported on their application forms that they had earned BS degrees in nursing, even though the requirement was that applicants needed only an associate's degree in nursing. Sarah hung her framed diploma on the wall by the receptionist desk. Christy has not brought her diploma in to be displayed. When she was asked to bring it in to hang by Sarah's diploma, Christy said that she had lost it in the move from Washington state to Alaska and just has not gotten around to replacing it.

Next month, Christy will have been employed at the clinic for one year. She is a good nurse; the doctors like her work; the patients like her compassionate manner; all like her pleasant personality. The office assistants have decided that a nice annual recognition to Christy would be to contact Christy's alma mater, purchase a duplicate diploma, frame it, and hang it for all to see. When the clinic manager contacts the university, she is informed that it has no record of Christy having graduated from their BS nursing program. It does, however, have a graduate by that name who received an associate's degree in nursing.

➤ Assume you are the clinic manager. Identify the problem in this case. What action, if any, should you take? What should you say, if anything, and to whom?

➤ Assume you are Sarah, the other nurse in the clinic. Identify the problem in this case. What action, if any, should you take? What should you say, if anything, and to whom?

➤ Assume you are one of the office assistants. Identify the problem in this case. What action, if any, should you take? What should you say, if anything, and to whom?

CHAPTER 9

DELEGATION

Community Hospital (CH) was trying something new. A large, downtown hospital, CH hoped to stream-line its patient discharge systems, increase its quality measures, and save money from its personnel budget by merging its discharge planning, social work, and patient advocacy offices. Chris Thompson, a social worker who had been with CH for about eight years, was asked to implement the change.

Chris was known for his meticulous work and attention to detail. He always said, "You have to be specific to be terrific." He prided himself on doing A+ work on his projects and for his patients. His bosses loved him because he not only did great work, but he also was willing to stay as long as necessary to get the job done. He could often be found at his desk long after hours, hand writing his patient notes until they were "just so."

Other than leading a number of smaller team projects over the years, this was Chris's first real management position, and he was determined to do it right and do it well. He had a vision for how the newly merged offices could work together more efficiently, and he was eager to dig in and make it happen.

He was a little surprised that even though everyone seemed to share his vision, they disagreed about how to get there. In fact, Chris was absolutely amazed at how little his colleagues agreed on. Meeting times were eaten up by arguments about how to arrange the desks in the offices, whether they should design their own department logo, and where to put the copy machine. Chris was so bogged down in trivial details that he started to lose sight of his vision of increased efficiency and harmony.

After his fourth plan for arranging the office space was shot down, he stomped into his office and closed his door. The day-to-day work still seemed to be getting done, but no progress had been made toward the real work of merging the offices.

Chris began preparing a PowerPoint presentation of his fifth proposal. He was still seeing his normal, pre-merger number of social work clients each week. He just hadn't had time to reassign his patients to other social workers or to bring his colleagues up to speed on his patients, many of whom had special circumstances and could not be handed off to other therapists without a fair amount of explanation.

Just that day, he'd gotten a memo from his boss asking him to create a pro forma budget for the upcoming management team meeting. That meant he'd have to go back into all three of last year's budgets for discharge planning, social work, and patient advocacy, pull out the information he needed, and then compile that information into a pro forma budget, whatever that was. He didn't know much about budgeting, and he wasn't very good at using the hospital's spreadsheet program. Still, he didn't want to ask the department secretary to do it, because she was swamped, too. He couldn't ask anyone else to do it; his colleagues were just as busy and probably didn't know anything about budgeting or using spreadsheets either. Anyway, if he asked for help, everyone would think that he didn't know what he was doing. He, who was perfect at *everything*.

LEARNING OBJECTIVES

After studying this chapter, you will be able to

➤ explain why it is often difficult to delegate,

➤ understand that delegation is a win-win technique for both the delegator and the delegatee, and

➤ outline the "Four Rights" approach to delegation.

9.1 DELEGATION CAN BE DIFFICULT

Chris' situation may sound contrived, but it is common in healthcare. Excellent caregivers moving up the relatively short career hierarchy soon find themselves in management positions—positions for which they have no training or experience. Yes, caregivers do manage their patients and lead care teams, but that is a different type of management from running or reorganizing a department or preparing budgets.

New managers coming up from the clinical side, like Chris, are not the only ones who have trouble delegating. Healthcare is an incredibly fast-paced environment, and work stacks up quickly for everyone. We look around, see everyone working at capacity, and can't imagine how we can possibly ask anyone to take on even one more task. So we do it ourselves. Chris's reluctance to ask his secretary to help him with spreadsheets is an example of this. For many healthcare managers, the volume of work simply becomes too much to handle, and **delegation** becomes a necessity rather than a luxury (Marquis and Huston 2000).

That said, it can be hard to let go of tasks. This is a feeling that many leaders share, As Ian Douglas Couper, MD (2007, 261), describes it:

> If I feel important, I start to do everything myself instead of delegating responsibilities. I fear passing tasks on to others because they will not do it the way I would or as well as I would (so I believe), but I become unable to do everything myself. I become an obstacle for myself and for others because I am doing too much. Delegation

Delegation
Assigning tasks to others; the ability to get work done through others.

is an important aspect of leadership and, distinct from off-loading work, it requires that I have a balanced view of myself. I sometimes believe that "my" hospital would collapse without me, yet it has continued to function at times when I was not there.

We can all relate to feeling that it is easier to do something yourself than to teach someone else how to do it. "It may seem that you can do the task better or faster than anyone else, but then you might be over-estimating the uniqueness of your skills and underestimating those of others. Clearly, if you don't break out of this trap there is a very real limit on what you can accomplish" (Culp and Smith 1997, 30).

When facing a new and difficult challenge, getting lost in those lower-level tasks where one feels comfortable can be soothing, as in the case of Chris and the furniture arrangements. People who climb the career ladder have been rewarded for their technical skills, knowledge, and task performance. As a result, many managers fear that delegating will diminish the importance of their own contributions in the eyes of their superiors or will be seen as a way to get out of doing the work themselves (Portny 2002). No one likes to look inadequate. Chris would rather figure out the pro forma budget and spreadsheet himself than admit to his colleagues that he doesn't know how to do it.

9.2 THE PLUS SIDE OF DELEGATION

According to an old joke, even God delegates. He asked Noah build the ark, and he had Moses lead the Israelites out of Egypt. Then Moses delegated some of his tasks to his brother Aaron, who was a better public speaker. One way of thinking about delegation, then, is that it is the ability to get work done through others (Curtis and Nicholl 2004; Kourdi 1999; Marquis and Huston 2000; Rocchiccioli and Tilbury 1998). Delegation extends results beyond what one person can do (Culp and Smith 1997). It enhances efficiency, time management, and productivity by distributing the work load (Ales 1995). And it frees managers to work on tasks for which they are better suited.

President Woodrow Wilson supposedly said, "I not only use all the brains I have, but all I can borrow." This provides another way to think about delegation. Done right, delegation can ensure that the most capable people available are working on the most appropriate tasks (Portny 2002). Delegation can allow employees to demonstrate their abilities, stretch, and learn new skills.

Delegation is not about finding a way to make your employees work harder so you have to do less work yourself. Delegation benefits the delegator and the delegatee. Delegators have more time for other managerial activities. They can focus on doing a few things well rather than too many things poorly. By delegating, they mentor and prepare employees for their own career advancement, resulting in higher-level performance. If work is done and decisions are made at the lowest appropriate level, everyone benefits from faster and more effective decision making.

Those to whom tasks are delegated have the opportunity to demonstrate their abilities, master new tasks, enhance their leadership and decision-making skills, gain a greater understanding of the work of the department and organization, network, and experience greater ownership over their work and the work of their colleagues.

9.3 DO YOU NEED TO DELEGATE MORE?

How does a manager know when she needs to delegate tasks? The signs may include the following (Culp and Smith 1997, 30):

- You work longer hours than your staff.

- You take work home regularly.

- You constantly rush to meet deadlines.

- You miss deadlines.

- You do or redo work that has been assigned to your staff.

- You regularly help with tasks you have delegated to others.

- Your own top-priority items remain undone.

- You are the only person you can identify as being able to handle the next big project.

- Your staff has low initiative.

- You have high turnover among your "rising stars."

9.4 WHAT TO DELEGATE AND WHAT NOT TO

Level of authority
An employee's ability to carry out delegated tasks. Levels include the authority to search for information, the authority to provide recommendations, and the authority to fully implement a task.

Delegation should not necessitate surrendering control of the process or of the outcome. Smart delegation is about giving employees the appropriate **level of authority** to carry out their assigned tasks (Kahn 2004). At the lowest level, an employee might be asked to look into a problem and to report back to the boss, who will then make the decision or take the action. A higher level of authority would involve the employee developing a recommendation, informing the boss about alternatives or pros and cons, and recommending a course of action. Even more authority would allow the employee to develop an action plan for the boss's approval. At the highest level, the boss might pass the authority to take action on to the employee and ask to be kept informed (Culp and Smith 1997).

9.5 THE FOUR RIGHTS APPROACH TO DELEGATION

Effective delegation takes thought, insight, and commitment. One way to simplify delegation is to use the **Four Rights approach**: the right task, the right person, the right communication, and the right feedback (Hantsen and Washburn 1992).

THE RIGHT TASK

Before delegating, the manager must accurately assess the work situation and environment. She must know the skills, abilities, interests, and limits of her employees. This doesn't mean she can only delegate a task to someone who already has the skill. Sometimes, a delegated task is an excellent opportunity for an employee to stretch and learn something new. The manager must have a grasp of her own skills and abilities and must know what responsibilities she should pass on to others and what tasks she should complete herself. She should beware of **dustbin delegation**—only delegating unpleasant, boring tasks that she just doesn't want to do herself. Delegated tasks should include enjoyable, appealing, and challenging tasks that are assigned according to skill and ability (Kourdi 1999).

THE RIGHT PERSON

Managers need to recognize the talents and personalities of their employees (Lewis 2000). "Choose a capable person, someone with intelligence, aptitude, and willingness to learn" (Culp and Smith 1997, 30). Matching the right person to the right task can be a challenge. Sometimes, the best way to pursue this is to look at each employee's "toolbox" and see whose background, previous work, and skills best fit the task at hand. Another option is to think about not only "who can do this," but also "who would enjoy this," or "who needs to acquire this particular skill," or "who is eager to stretch."

THE RIGHT COMMUNICATION

Assignments need to be clear and well defined. "Successful delegation includes information on what, when, who, and, perhaps, how. The employee must clearly understand the task and the expected results" (Daft 1991, 253). It is best to stress desired outcomes, not details or methods of production (Lewis 2000). "Point out the potential failure paths and what not to do, but don't specify every detail of how to do the task. Identify the human, financial, technical, and organizational resources the person can draw on to accomplish the desired results" (Covey 1990, 174). Agree upon the standards for performance that will be used to evaluate the results, a timeline, and the deliverables. Last, specify what will happen—good and bad—as a result of the evaluation of the task.

Four Rights approach
Delegating by assigning the right task, the right person, the right communication, and the right feedback.

Dustbin delegation
Delegating only unpleasant, boring tasks that the manager doesn't want to have to do.

THE RIGHT FEEDBACK

Throughout the project, keep the lines of communication open. Establish checkpoints and provide objective feedback. If the delegated task is not moving ahead as it should, address your concerns promptly; don't allow the task to go completely awry. It can be difficult to provide negative feedback, but allowing the employee to continue down a path of inappropriate or unsatisfactory progress helps no one. Provide negative feedback in private, and try to address the ineffective behavior or poor outcomes. Discuss specific, objective details, and ask the employee to provide alternatives for improvement.

If the task is on target, provide praise as appropriate. Be certain to deliver any agreed-upon rewards. Give credit where credit is due; a manager who takes the credit for his employees' good work will not be respected and will have difficulty delegating in the future.

9.6 DO YOU HAVE A PROBLEM DELEGATING?

The following list of questions relate to a manager's attitudes and perspectives. If you answer yes to more than three of these questions, you may have a problem with delegating.

- ◆ I tend to be a perfectionist.

- ◆ My boss expects me to know all the details of my job.

- ◆ I don't have the time to explain clearly and concisely how a task should be accomplished.

- ◆ I often end up doing tasks myself.

- ◆ My subordinates typically are not as committed as I am.

- ◆ I get upset when other people don't do the task right.

- ◆ I really enjoy doing the details of my job to the best of my ability.

- ◆ I like to be in control of task outcomes.

(Daft 1991, 253)

9.7 CHRIS AND THE NEWLY MERGED DEPARTMENT

When Chris's boss realized that Chris was in over his head with the newly merged department, she suggested that Chris answer the eight questions listed above. Chris answered yes to each question. As a result, he realized that he needed to adjust his attitudes and activities. He needed to stop trying to make everyone happy with furniture arrangements and begin the work of merging the three departments into one. He needed to learn how to delegate.

DISCUSSION QUESTIONS

➤ Chris needs to take a step back and create a plan for merging the department that in-cludes the delegation of appropriate tasks to his employees. Which tasks do you think will be easiest for Chris to delegate? Which will be the most difficult?

➤ Review the list of questions concerning work situations that imply a need to start dele-gating. Which of these are alive and well in your current work situation?

➤ Refer to the list of attitudes and perceptions near the end of this chapter. Which of these do you hold? Why? How can these attitudes and perceptions be double-edged swords?

EXERCISE 9.1   "YOU'VE GOT E-MAIL AND A SURPRISE"

Donna Bourkovski, a marketing manager at Southern Pines Hospital in North Carolina, has just returned from her vacation. She and her family visited Yellowstone National Park, and Donna has not opened her laptop for two weeks. She knew that when she returned to her desk, she would have to do a great deal of work just to catch up. But she had enjoyed the nat-ural landscape of America's first national park. She saw wolves, a brown bear, and several buf-falo. She and her family hiked, fished in the streams, and saw Old Faithful erupt several times. But now it is time to return to work, and Donna has arrived early to respond to e-mails.

Southern Pines Hospital is a 300-bed facility located between two cities, and it offers services to the residents of both. It serves as the center for clinic placements for Southern North Carolina State University. Donna has served as the marketing manager for five years, and she knows how the public relations and marketing department works. She hopes that she will be promoted to vice president of public relations and marketing at some point. She enjoys work-ing for and learning from her supervisor at Southern Pines Hospital, Elwood O'Toole. He is knowledgeable, funny, and full of surprises. He has been a good mentor to her, and Donna thinks that when he decides to retire, he might consider recommending her for the position. She expects he will retire in the next year, as he is in his late sixties and has mentioned that he and his wife want to spend more time together and travel while they are still in good health.

It is 6:30 a.m. on Monday, August 4, and Donna is in her office. She will be meeting with Elwood at 7:15 to review what has occurred during her absence and to receive new in-structions. Donna has 45 minutes to go through her e-mail and respond appropriately. She wants to get this work done so she is ready to address whatever Elwood assigns to her. In responding to the e-mails, she needs to be sure that she returns e-mails and writes memos or instructions as appropriate. For this exercise, take the role of Donna. You have 45 minutes to address the following e-mails appropriately. Your work should be completed within the 45-minute time frame.

Donna's E-mails

To: Donna
From: Elwood
RE: Retirement
Date: 8/1

Nice to have you back, Donna. As your supervisor, I am letting you know first that my wife and I have decided that it is time for me to retire. I want to talk with you this morning about your applying for the position of vice president of public relations and marketing. In the meantime, I am asking you to serve as the interim VP. I assume you will say yes, so I have taken the liberty of attaching a few things that might be helpful as you serve as Interim VP. Attached you will find:

1. The new organizational chart
2. Some notes on public relations/marketing employees based upon annual reviews and personal observations

---

FIGURE 9.1
Southern Pines
Hospital
Organizational
Chart

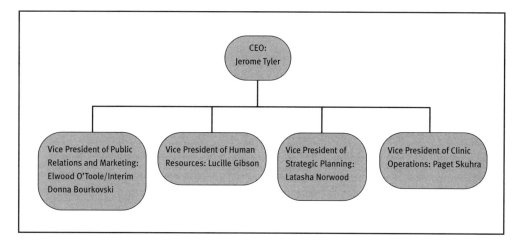

TABLE 9.1
Notes on Employees

Name	Position	Remarks
Mary Brookes	Public Relations Coordinator	Inconsistent performer; three years at hospital. Recommended to take communications seminar to improve presentation skills (5/2).
Yolanda Buchanan	Administrative Assistant to VP of Public Relations and Marketing	Solid, consistent performer; 18 years at the hospital.
Diane Wilson	Marketing Consultant	Receives outstanding annual evaluations. Top performer with the public; stays calm and handles communication crises well; knows television reporters as she left the local TV station to take on this job; 30 years in the department.

To: Donna
From: Vice Presidents
RE: Welcome
Date: 8/1

Elwood told us that you are the Interim VP. Congratulations! Glad you are on board with us, Donna. The other VPs are looking forward to spending some time with you. How about you and your husband joining us at the university preseason football scrimmage this Saturday (8/9)? Tailgating is hosted by Jerome Tyler. See you then.

To: All VPs
From: Lucille
RE: HR Timecard Training
Date: 8/1

HR online timecard training must be completed by Thursday! Make sure you attend one of the training sessions offered by HR. Training dates/times are: Monday at noon, Tuesday at 5 p.m., and Wednesday at 8 a.m.

To: Donna B.
From: Lucille
Date: 8/1
RE: Job Reassignments

Elwood told me you are the interim VP. I am very happy that you are working in this position. I've thought about Elwood's request to grant his secretary, Yolanda Buchanan, a reassignment because of an ADA issue. Please take care of this.

To: Donna
Forwarded from Elwood 8/1
From: Paget
Re: Customer Complaints
Date: 7/7

I received a letter this morning from a community member who complained about the way his granddaughter was treated by the public relations coordinator, Mary Brookes, at the Big Sister training at our Family Birthing Center. This is the second complaint I have received about community relations mishaps. What is going on with your community education programs? Can you handle this?

To: All VPs
From: Latasha
Date: 8/1
RE: Meeting

Reminder: Strategic planning meeting at the East Campus Conference Room at 9 a.m. on August 19.

To: Donna
Forwarded from Elwood 8/3
From: Lucille
RE: Complaint
Date: 6/30

Your marketing consultant Diane Wilson has complained of age discrimination. Can you handle this?

To: Donna
Forwarded from Elwood 8/3
From: Jerome
RE: Employees' names, positions, years at Southern Pines
Date: 6/30

Elwood, I need a list of your employees' names, positions, and years worked at Southern Pines. I want to recognize the workers at our Kick Off for the Annual Fund Drive in September.

To: All VPs
Forwarded from Elwood 8/3
From: Latasha
RE: Strategic Plans from Last Year
Date: 5/14

Please e-mail me a copy of last year's strategic plan. I will use this information for our meeting to be held in August.

To: Donna
From: Diane
RE: Meeting
Date: 7/30

Hello, Donna. I want to talk with you about something that is going on at work. When you get back from your vacation, let's set up a time to meet, okay? Thanks.

To: Donna
From: Yolanda
RE: Asthma
Date: 7/23

Donna, there is a problem with the new air conditioning system in our offices. I will be working at the module because I am having difficulty breathing in our current office. My e-mail address stays the same, of course, but I do have a new phone number, extension 2842.

➤ Did you find that you wanted to put off some of the work and address it later? Why or why not is this appropriate for the e-mails listed?

➤ Review your decisions. Were there any actions you could have delegated to an appropriate person that you chose to do yourself?

EXERCISE 9.2 JOY'S COMPLAINT

Suzzie Brennecke has been the clinic manager for the Medgroup Management Practice in Nashville, Tennessee, for 12 years. She is responsible for all staff and business operations in the practice. The practice is made up of three dermatologists, two plastic surgeons, and three nurses. Minor surgeries are conducted on the premises. It is Suzzie's responsibility to ensure that the office runs smoothly, patients' calls are received promptly, medical records are in order, billing is conducted on a timely and regular basis, and materials and equipment are ordered and stored properly.

Suzzie is also responsible for all personnel issues. She hires, motivates, evaluates, and sometimes fires employees. Suzzie finds that she is constantly hiring office assistants, as turnover is higher than at comparable practices. She finds herself working late to review the billing system for which Joy, the billing officer, is responsible. Joy has worked at the practice for two years and is very comfortable with her ability to bill appropriately. She knows the coding procedures and she has a good record regarding billing collections. She has asked why Suzzie stays late to review her billing work all the time, or to do work that other assistants could do during the day.

Joy says, "Suzzie, my work is excellent. Do you really think you need to review my efforts on such a regular basis? You are busy. If you want to review, why don't you ask Linda to help? She has been working in the practice for almost nine months now, and she has been asking for more responsibility in the office. All she does is answer the phones, and she would like to have more variety."

Suzzie responds, "Joy, I am ultimately responsible for all operations in the practice. I need to conduct the review."

Joy tries again. "Suzzie, I don't want to lose Linda. She has a lot of talent, and she is getting bored doing the same task over and over. You are overworked. Can't you allow us to take on some of jobs you do?"

Suzzie waves away Joy with shake of her head. "Oh, Joy, I need to do it."

The next week, Linda resigns from the Medgroup Management Practice. Suzzie sighs to herself, "Now I have to go out and hire somebody else. I don't understand why Linda is leaving us. She was very competent and Joy was right—she had a lot of talent. Oh well, I need to move forward with writing the advertisement and putting it in the paper and on the website. Then I'll need to interview. Nobody else can handle this."

➤ Do you think Suzzie is a good practice manager? Why or why not?

➤ Consider the signs that Daft (1991) lists regarding difficulty delegating. Does Suzzie seem to have difficulty with delegating?

➤ With the information provided, how can Suzzie become a better practice manager? What would you recommend she do to retain good staff members at the practice?

CHAPTER 10

HIRING, MOTIVATING, EVALUATING, AND TERMINATING STAFF

CASE STUDY PROFESSIONAL BEHAVIOR

Dr. Dorothy Daunt, chair of the Medical University biology department, had just met with Roberta Smith, a nursing student. Over 12,000 students, all preparing for careers in medicine, attend the university, and all are required to take Dr. Charles Fox's course, Cell Biology. The students are studying to become physical therapists, occupational therapists, radiology technologists, physicians, nurses, pharmacists, etc.

Over 200 cell slides are shown per class in Dr. Fox's course, and the students need to remember each slide. Dr. Fox slips in an X-rated slide—always a nude woman—before he shows "important" slides.

Roberta Smith has objected to this practice. She spoke to the professor and requested that he use different surprise slides. She recommended using baby pictures or people snow-skiing on the slopes or impressive sunset panoramas. However, Dr. Fox defended his practice by saying that the nude pictures work. "They get the students' attention, and the students will remember what a real cancer slide looks like." Roberta met with Dr. Daunt and explained that she found the pictures of nude women offensive and intimidating. "How would you like to be trying to memorize what a cancer cell looks like when the professor pops in a slide like that? I sometimes get a stomachache just thinking about having to come to class." She asked Dr. Daunt to stop Dr. Fox from showing the nude slides in class.

Dr. Daunt promised Roberta that she would follow up. After Roberta left the office, Dr. Daunt called the university's human resources and legal departments. She wanted to review university policy regarding such behavior before she spoke with Dr. Fox. She was concerned that the professor might be in violation of sexual harassment laws. Last, she pulled Dr. Fox's file and noted that his annual reviews were positive. He had been in her department for two years, and she knew him to have an excellent publication record. His research area was pancreatic cancer and pain management, and his work was nationally recognized. His service work to the cancer community was exemplary. She knew little about his teaching, but had heard comments that some students did not like him. The phone rang for her conference call with Legal and HR. As she picked up the receiver, she wondered why some intelligent people showed little sense. She knew that showing nude pictures in class was not right. How had the Medical University gotten stuck with this guy?

LEARNING OBJECTIVES

After studying this chapter, you will be able to

➤ appreciate the significance of organizational fit in hiring,

➤ identify the job description document and explore its role in the hiring process,

➤ identify retention and discuss current retention issues in healthcare organizations,

➤ describe the performance evaluation process,

➤ understand the HR termination process and consider key factors involved in the process, and

➤ understand the issue of sexual harassment in the workplace.

10.1 HIRING THE BEST FIT

Two critical factors for healthcare managers to consider during the hiring process are (1) the need to hire a person qualified for the position advertised and (2) the need to hire someone who will perform well in the specific work environment. Building a team of staff members who possess the knowledge, skills, and abilities to do their jobs well and who work well together allows a department to perform well. The goal of recruitment is to find the person who meets the specific job requirements and who is the best **organizational fit**. Dr. Fox may be an excellent researcher and may be highly involved with professional service; however, his behavior as a teacher may not fit well in his specific work environment.

Fottler (2001) proposed that a **job description** may be used to clearly define the tasks, duties, responsibilities, and performance standards associated with the position. The use of a job description may enhance the candidate's awareness of expectations pertaining to the specific job requirements. The following box gives the job description for Dr. Fox's position. The description clearly states that the professor is expected to teach, conduct research, and participate in professional service. Specific to Roberta's concern, the description also states that the professor is expected to exhibit professional behavior.

Organizational fit

An employment candidate's qualification for the position advertised and ability to work well with others in the specific work environment.

Job description

A document that clearly defines the tasks, duties, responsibilities, and performance standards associated with a position.

<table>
<tr><td>

(✳) JOB DESCRIPTION

Position: Assistant Professor, Biology, Medical University

Specifications: Assistant Professor, Tenure Track, Department of Biology, College of Health Professions, Medical University. The professor is expected to possess exceptional communication skills and exhibit professional behavior. PhD in cell biology preferred. The assistant professor will be expected to

1. teach six credit hours per semester in the Department of Biology to large classes of health-profession students,
2. engage in scholarly research, and
3. participate in professional service activities at the local, state, and/or national levels.

</td></tr>
</table>

Bowen, Ledford, and Nathan (1991) support the practice of hiring based on a candidate's good fit with the organization as well as his good fit for the position. That is, the candidate should have the credentials and knowledge for the position, but he should also possess qualities that are in sync with the organizational culture. With reference to the hiring of Dr. Fox, the question emerges of whether behavioral expectations should have been emphasized more during the interview process. Alternatively, the hiring team could have underscored the importance of fit with the organization. However, even if the hiring team had emphasized a culture of professionalism, Dr. Fox still might have exhibited the behavior Roberta described. No hiring system is perfect.

Nonetheless, the takeaway from Bowen, Ledford, and Nathan's (1991) research is the importance of a good fit between individual and job and between individual and organization. There are advantages for the person and for the organization to selecting candidates whose values fit with the organization's culture. These advantages include higher reported job satisfaction (Kristof 1996; Adkins and Caldwell 2004), positive work performance (Kristof 1996; Hoffman and Woehr 2006), and lower turnover (Chatman 1991; O'Reilly, Chatman, and Caldwell 1991).

A hiring misstep may result in extra work and additional stress for the manager and the other staff members throughout the person's employment. The manager must also spend more of her time on corrective action plans and disciplinary options. In the case study, Dr. Daunt met with Roberta and arranged for the meeting with the HR and legal departments. She will be meeting with Dr. Fox, arranging for follow through with regard to Dr. Fox's response, and supervising Dr. Fox's in-class behavior. If Roberta files a formal complaint with the EEO/Affirmative Action office on campus, Dr. Daunt could be involved in an EEO hearing. She is spending and will spend more time and effort because a member of her team is behaving questionably.

This incident could have positive outcomes. If Dr. Fox were to understand that the slide show is unacceptable, he may learn from his mistake and become a better teacher. As he is excellent with research and service, certainly this outcome is possible. Part of Dr. Daunt's responsibilities as chair is to supervise and lead the departmental members to become better professionals. This incident provides an excellent opportunity for Dr. Daunt to guide Dr. Fox. However, Dr. Daunt is currently questioning how the university "got stuck" with Dr. Fox.

Steps to determine whether a qualified candidate also demonstrates fit with the organization include the following:

1. Review the position advertisement and job description.

2. Screen applicant files to ensure each candidate's qualifications meet the job specifications.

3. Participate in the interview process.

4. Evaluate each candidate's strengths and weaknesses.

5. Contact each candidate's references.

6. Advise the administration regarding candidate selection preferences.

7. Continually work with an HR representative throughout the process.

Another important factor is training about an appropriate hiring process. When the hiring team is conducting interviews, they should know what they can and cannot ask a candidate. They may ask questions about a candidate's past job and educational experiences and questions regarding the candidate's ability to perform the specific job advertised. They may not ask questions about the candidate's age (unless the specific job has an age requirement), family status (married, divorced, single, parent, etc.), credit status, handicaps unrelated to job performance, political affiliation, race, or religion. The purpose of the applicant screening is to ascertain whether the applicant meets the job qualifications. The purpose of the face-to-face interview is to allow the recruiting team members to meet candidates, and vice versa. The candidate can use this time to assess whether the organization is a good fit for him. Given that employees will spend at least 40 hours per week at a job, good fit is important to the organization and to the candidate.

A challenge specific to hiring in the healthcare industry is the current healthcare labor shortage. Sportsman (2007) describes it as a challenge of finding and retaining competent people during a shortage of competent healthcare professionals. The healthcare industry is experiencing and will continue to experience a shortage of nurses, pharmacists, technicians, and therapists (Coile 2002). The shortages exacerbate the challenge. Recruitment teams seek the best person with the best fit for the position, but find themselves in a highly competitive environment. As a result, healthcare organization managers who are able to hire people should also be concerned about keeping the people they have hired. Griffith and White (2007) note that it is less costly to an organization to retain (for example) nurses than it is to recruit new nurses.

10.2 RETENTION AND PERFORMANCE APPRAISALS: THE IMPORTANCE OF FEEDBACK

Retention

The keeping of employees at an organization.

Retention refers to keeping good staff at an organization. Turnover is costly in terms of the time spent to replace a staff member and the dollars spent to advertise, review applications, and interview candidates. Effective managers should look into why good staff members leave an organization, and what encourages them to stay. The reasons someone leaves an organization may highlight what can be done to keep other valued employees. Donoghue and Castle (2007) found that LPNs, RNs, and NAs often left their positions in nursing homes because of work environment. Understaffing and the organizations' deficiency citations were reported as the primary reasons.

The Joint Commission

A not-for-profit accrediting agency that assesses an organizations' ability to meet standards of performance in key healthcare operations.

Managers have an ongoing responsibility to hire the most competent and committed healthcare professionals. However, with the current labor shortage, this responsibility has become a challenge. Hence, employee retention is essential to organizational success. **The Joint Commission** assesses healthcare organizations according to standards of performance in key healthcare operations (such as infection control, patient treatment, etc). The Joint Commission is a not-for-profit accrediting agency that currently reviews hospitals; home care organizations; hospices; long-term care facilities; behavioral healthcare, substance abuse, and mental health programs; ambulatory care centers; and independent laboratories. The review is focused on quality assurance, and The Joint Commission's mission is to "continuously improve the safety and quality of care provided to the public through the provision of healthcare accreditation and related services that support performance improvement in healthcare organizations" (The Joint Commission 2008). Creating and sustaining a work environment that focuses on providing a well-staffed healthcare organization meeting The Joint Commission's standards is key for retention. Other characteristics of retention strategies include

1.   a focus on the positive recognition of staff members' accomplishments,

2.   a compensation process that is linked to staff members' work performance,

3. a culture of mutual respect,

4. a competitive package that includes leave time for vacation and holidays,

5. opportunities for professional training and development,

6. a commitment by leaders to provide the resources necessary to meet accreditation agencies' standards, and

7. a commitment by managers to implement the organization's retention strategy.

Gering and Conner (2002) propose that the best managers follow a strategy that values their employees, meets employees' personal and practical needs (i.e., salary, work schedule, vacation time), provides rewards and recognition when appropriate, allows for professional advancement, provides compelling reasons the employees should be a part of the organization, and links compensation with **performance evaluation**. The Institute of Management and Administration (**IOMA**) conducts an annual survey of businesses to assess human resource issues and track compensation trends. The 2007 survey indicated that almost half of the firms with more than 7,000 employees paid top performers more than low performers, while about a third of the firms with 199 or fewer employees did so. Linking performance to pay is related to lower turnover of top performers, as the employees see first-hand that merit matters.

Performance evaluations can be formal or informal. A simple acknowledgment of an employee's work is informal. "Nice, the way you were able to explain that procedure to the new technician today," is an example of informal, immediate feedback. Feedback is critical to providing leadership, maintaining contact, and assessing staff members' understanding of their work. Gratto Liebler and McConnell (2008) recommend that managers remain in regular contact with each employee. The interactions allow managers and employees to identify and address potential problems and provide a manager with opportunities to notice and an employee with a chance to hear about work well done.

Formal performance evaluations are performed on a regular basis. Typically, they are held annually with each staff member to provide feedback regarding performance and performance standards and to offer guidance for the employee's goals for the upcoming year. Effective performance evaluations include overall assessment of the employee's strengths and weaknesses, recommendations for improvement in performance, and information that is the basis for compensation, promotions, or corrective actions. Figure 10.1 is an example of a performance appraisal used by Portneuf Medical Center (PMC). It includes an assessment of the employee's progress toward the goals made at the previous year's review and identifies the employee's plan for the upcoming year. Furthermore, it provides information to which the manager may refer when making promotion and salary decisions.

Performance evaluation
The process whereby the work behavior and efforts of employees are reviewed.

IOMA
The Institute of Management and Administration, a professional organization for managers.

FIGURE 10.1

PMC Performance Appraisal Form Example: CFO's Annual Review

 Portneuf
MEDICAL CENTER
Where Care and Compassion Reside

PORTNEUF MEDICAL CENTER
LEADERSHIP POSITION DESCRIPTION/PERFORMANCE EVALUATION

Job Title:	Department Name:	Evaluation period:	
Employee Name:	Employee Signature: *(My signature acknowledges that the information below has been discussed with me and that I have had the opportunity to add my comments to this review.)*		Date:
Manager Name:	Manager Signature:		Date:

PERFORMANCE RATING SYSTEM DEFINITIONS

0- Unsatisfactory – Performance falls below expected levels. Performance is **not at supervisor's expectations**. Individual unable and/or unwilling to meet job expectations. Improvement must be made in order to meet full expectations of the job. Performance requires an immediate action plan.

1- Growth Opportunity – Needs Improvement. Occasionally **inconsistent or unreliable** performance. The employee may have a basic understanding of the job responsibilities, but is unable to perform this standard without additional assistance, monitoring, or training. Performance is acceptable some of the time, and further improvement is needed.

2- Consistently meets performance standards. Successful level of performance **as expected**. The employee at this level has a complete understanding of the position, requires minimal supervision and consistently performs all aspects of the job responsibilities

3- Commendable. Performance is consistently **above and beyond** all expectations. The employee is continually working on personal development and achieves personal goals. Relates well to all kinds of people and builds constructive and effective relationships and is seen as a role model to co-workers.

4- Outstanding. Highest level of observed performance marked by **extraordinary achievements** when compared to expected performance. Performance at this level **substantially exceeds** all aspects of the job responsibilities. Eliminates roadblocks, creates focus, and makes good decisions based upon a mixture of analysis, wisdom, experience, and judgment. The employee acts as a resource for both the management and staff in originating new ways of doing things and uses this influence to guide the work group/department to levels that otherwise would not be reached. Characteristic of 5-10% of employees.

Note:
> * Any item rated as "Outstanding", "Growth Opportunity", or "Unsatisfactory", requires a Manager comment.
> * Any item rated as "Unsatisfactory" requires a plan for improvement. List in goals section.
> * An overall score of "less than 2.00" requires a Performance Improvement Plan. Please attach.

LEADERSHIP CORE COMPETENCIES			
LEADERSHIP CATEGORY	**EVALUATION / COMMENTS**	**RATING**	**AVERAGE**
To compute the average rating for each category, please right click on the average and select 'Update Field'.			
Leadership: *Focuses and guides others in accomplishing work objectives* 1. Sets specific performance goals and identifies measures for evaluating goal achievement		0	
2. Identifies specific behaviors, knowledge, and skill areas for focus and evaluation.		0	0.00
3. Holds regular discussions with direct reports to discuss progress towards goals.		0	
4. Consistently follows established center wide policies and processes.		0	
Develop Relationships: *Interacts with others in a way that gives them confidence in one's intentions and those of the organization; develops and uses collaborative relationships to facilitate the accomplishment of work goals.* 1. Proactively works to build effective working relationships.		0	
2. Listens to others and objectively considers others' ideas and opinions, even when they conflict with their own.		0	0.00
3. Treats people with dignity, respect and fairness; gives proper credit to others; stands up for deserving others and their ideas even in the face of resistance or challenge.		0	
Integrity: *Maintains social, ethical, and organizational norms; firmly adheres to mission, vision and values, service excellence standards of behavior, codes of conduct and ethical principles.* 1. Deals with people in an honest and forthright manner		0	0.00
2. Represents information and data accurately and completely.		0	
3. Performs actions as promised.		0	
4. Does not share confidential information.		0	

FIGURE 10.1

PMC Performance
Appraisal Form
Example: CFO's
Annual Review
(continued)

5. Ensures that words and actions are consistent.		0	
6. Understands the internal and external processes available to all employees for reporting any accreditation, HIPAA, or legal concerns, and that there shall be no retaliatory action taken toward any employee for any reason related to reporting such a concern. *(Employee should note any concerns that they wish to report at this time under employee comments.)*		0	
Team Building: *Uses appropriate methods and a flexible interpersonal style; helps build a cohesive team; facilitating the completion of team goals.* 1. Ensures that the purpose and importance of the team are clarified (e.g., team has a clear purpose).		0	
2. Guides the setting of specific and measurable team goals and objectives.		0	0.00
3. Helps to clarify roles and responsibilities of team members.		0	
4. Provides necessary resources or helps to remove obstacles team accomplishments.		0	
5. Listens to and fully involves others in team decisions and actions in a way that values all.		0	
Strategic Perspective: *Obtains information and identifies key issues and relationships relevant to a long-range goal or vision; commits to a course of action to accomplish a long-range goal or vision after developing alternatives based on logical assumptions, facts available resources, constraints, and organizational values.* 1. Demonstrates an understanding of the underlying forces driving our industry and/or areas of discipline.		0	
2. Stays abreast of internal and external industry events to help formulate decision-making criteria.		0	0.00
3. Makes judgments and decision in light of strategy.		0	

System Thinking: *Understands the complexity and interrelatedness of functions, departments, processes, actions and decisions on producing desired outcomes for the organization.* 1. Demonstrates and understands consequences of decisions, involves others in problem solving; sees the connections throughout the organization.		0	
2. Thinks issues through beyond the immediate.		0	0.00
3. Appreciates the impact of actions on other areas.		0	
4. Has a sophisticated view of the relationships between organizational levels.		0	
5. Understands how decisions affect the work of others.		0	
Manage Performance: *Assesses staff effectiveness and development needs on a regular basis; confronts negative behavior to foster acceptance and change; provides honest feedback and provide recognition for a job well done.* 1. Clarifies expected behaviors, knowledge and level of proficiency by seeking and giving information and checking for understanding.		0	
2. Gives timely, appropriate feedback on performance; reinforces efforts and progress.		0	0.00
3. Recognizes poor performance and deals with it in a timely manner.		0	
4. Establishes good interpersonal relationships by helping people feel valued, appreciated and included.		0	
5. Ensures that appropriate opportunities for development are available.		0	
Safety: *Identifies and corrects conditions that affect employee and patient safety; upholding safety and environment of care standards.* 1. Detects hazardous conditions and safety problems.		0	0.00
2. Makes recommendations and/or improves safety and security procedures.		0	
3. Provides appropriate training.		0	

FIGURE 10.1

PMC Performance
Appraisal Form
Example: CFO's
Annual Review
(continued)

4. Monitors safety or security issues after taking corrective action and ensures continued compliance.		0	
Trust and Respect: *Interacts with others in a way that gives them confidence in their intentions and those of the organization.* 1. Operates with integrity. Demonstrates honesty; keeps commitments; behaves in a consistent manner.		0	**0.00**
2. Remains open to ideas Listens to others and objectively considers other's ideas and opinions, even when they conflict with their own.		0	
Decision Making: *Identifies and understands issues, problems, and opportunities; compares data from different sources to draw conclusions. Uses effective approaches for choosing a course of action or developing appropriate solutions; commits to an action after developing alternative courses of action based on logical assumptions and factual information—taking into consideration, resources constraints, and organizational values.* 1. Recognizes issues, problems or opportunities and determines whether action is needed.		0	
2. Identifies the need for and collects information to better understand issues; problems and opportunities.		0	
3. Integrates information from a variety of sources; detects trends, associations and cause-effect relationships.		0	**0.00**
4. Formulates clear decision criteria; evaluates options by considering implications and consequences; chooses an effective option.		0	
5. Implements decisions or initiates action within a reasonable time.		0	
6. Includes others in the decision-making process as warranted to obtain good information, make the most appropriate decisions and ensure by-in and understanding of the resulting decisions.		0	

Delegation: *Allocates decision-making authority and/or task responsibility to appropriate others to maximize the organizations and individuals effectiveness.* 1. Allocates decision-making authority and/or task responsibility in appropriate areas to appropriate individuals (considering positive and negative impact, organizational values and structures and the enhancement of the individual's knowledge and skills).		0	
2. Clearly communicates the parameters of the delegated responsibility, including decision-making authority and any required actions, constraints, or deadlines.		0	**0.00**
3. Suggests resources and provides assistance or coaching as needed; expresses confidence in the individual.		0	
4. Establishes appropriate procedures to keep informed of issues and results in areas of shared responsibility.		0	
Leadership Competencies Average Weighted Score (70%)	*To compute the Average Weighted Score, please right click on the formula and select 'update field'.*		**0.00**

POSITION DESCRIPTION			
POSITION PURPOSE: The incumbent must be a seasoned manager who is well organized, self-directed and capable of a broad range of managerial tasks. Daily activities will include planning, organizing and implementing strategies, as well as effective delegation and mentoring in a participative environment. The incumbent must be approachable and give useful feedback to staff regarding their job performance. As the organization continues to change, difficult decisions will need to be made, requiring a high degree of judgment, tact, and the ability to lead by example.			
JOB SPECIFIC RESPONSIBILITIES	**EVALUATION METHOD**	**EVALUATION / COMMENTS**	**RATING**

FIGURE 10.1
PMC Performance
Appraisal Form
Example: CFO's
Annual Review
(continued)

Develops a budget to ensure adequate resources are allocated in support of department programs and priorities. Develops capital, operating, and salary budgets annually and maintains budgets within approved limits. Monitors and interprets monthly financial statements, taking corrective action in response to variances and trends.	Observation Audits Reports		0
Ensures there is adequate staffing to meet the needs of the daily operations. On bi-weekly basis, reviews employee time cards for hours worked and approves for payment of wages based on current compensation and/or benefit policies.	Observation Audits Reports		0
Ensures that staff is continuously trained to provide competent care through development, implementation, and ongoing support of appropriate, competency based orientation, education, and evaluation programs.	Observation Audits Reports		0
Possesses broad-based knowledge in their profession. Demonstrates the ability to quickly understand key issues and priorities within their area of accountability. Continually stays abreast of trends in their field of expertise, demonstrating a commitment to continuing education, both on a personal level, and in supporting and assessing staff members' needs for continuing education.	Observation Audits Reports		0
Develops and maintains a department quality/performance improvement plan consistent with the Center's program. Applies performance improvement (PI) principles to all appropriate operating systems.	Observation Audits Reports		0
Operates effectively within the applicable constraints imposed by state and federal legal statutes, JCAHO requirements, and requirements of other external agencies as appropriate.	Observation Audits Reports		0
Job Responsibilities Average Weighted Score (20%)	*To compute the Average Weighted Score, please right click on the formula and select 'update field'.*		**0.00**

MINIMUM QUALIFICATIONS

Requirements are representative of minimum level of knowledge, skills, and/or abilities.

Licensure/Education Qualifications:
For effective performance in this position, the incumbent must possess: thorough knowledge and understanding of accounting principles and practices; strong management capabilities; effective communication skills; judgment, tact, and diplomacy; strong interpersonal abilities; computer and software skills; and effective organizational skills. This combination of knowledge and skills typically would be acquired through the following:

1. Bachelor's degree in Accounting or closely related field.
2. CPA Licensure preferred.
3. Three years or more of background in the accounting field, preferably in a health care setting. Two years of management experience.

Physical Requirements:
While performing the duties of this job, the employee is regularly required to sit; stand; walk; use hands to finger, handle or feel; reach with hands and arms; and rarely stoop, kneel, crouch, or crawl. Occasionally required to climb, and lift/carry up to 15 pounds. Works in office areas, as well as throughout the facility. Interacts with other staff, visitors, family members, sales persons, and physicians under many conditions and circumstances. May be subject to hostile and emotionally upset patients and other individuals. Drives frequently between two sites that are approximately a mile and a half apart.

Working Environment:

ORGANIZATIONAL EXPECTATIONS

STRATEGIC GOALS 2007-2011:

1. **AVAILABILITY OF CARE**

   Portneuf Medical Center will improve availability of healthcare services throughout Eastern Idaho.

2. **INFORMATION SYSTEMS**

   Portneuf Medical Center will implement its information system strategic plan and move toward a single electronic patient medical record.

3. **MARKET SHARE / REGIONAL REFERRAL CENTER**

   Portneuf Medical Center will grow its market share in the region and become the regional leader in medical referral relationships from the surrounding region.

4. **OPERATIONAL EXCELLENCE**

   Portneuf Medical Center will achieve recognizable operational excellence in its overall operation of the Medical Center.

5. **ORGANIZATIONAL INTEGRATION**

   Portneuf Medical Center will be integrated into a single campus and cohesive organization.

FIGURE **10.1**
PMC Performance
Appraisal Form
Example: CFO's
Annual Review
(continued)

MISSION STATEMENT

❖   Portneuf Medical Center provides compassionate, quality health care services needed by the people of Eastern Idaho in collaboration with other providers and community resources.

VISION STATEMENT

❖   By 2012, Portneuf Medical Center will be a single campus regional referral center with well-defined centers of excellence, serving Eastern Idaho.

VALUES STATEMENT

❖   These beliefs and values are the foundation of our mission and vision:

- Compassion   - We care for others as if they are members of our own family.
- Dignity - We treat every person with respect.
- Excellence - We continually improve our services to ensure the highest quality of care.
- Education - We maintain a commitment to growth and learning.
- Accountability – We use resources wisely to ensure that services are consistently provided at appropriate cost.
- Collaboration – We work with others to improve the health status of the community.

TEAM / PERSONAL GOALS	RATING
ACCOMPLISHMENTS/CONTRIBUTIONS *(Include a review of the previous year's individual goals and date completed.)*	0
Team/Personal Goals Weighted Score (10%) / *To compute the Weighted Score, please right click on the formula and select 'update field'.*	0.00

INDIVIDUAL GOALS FOR NEXT YEAR *- (To be completed by Employee and their Supervisor.)*
In this section, list specific job-related goals & objectives for the next twelve months. These work-related goals link to the strategic goals by directly supporting your department's goals. These goals should include those relating to your primary job responsibilities, key initiates, and projects. **At least two goals are required.**

SUPPORT What Strategic Goal do your goals support?	SPECIFIC List specifically what goals you will accomplish	MEASURABLE How will you know they are completed?	ATTAINABLE & REALISTIC Are the goals realistic and can they completed within the next year?	TIMEFRAME Dates the goals will be completed

CORE COMPETENCY & MANDATORY EDUCATION
Were all requirements completed within specified timeframe?
Completed all Annual mandatory education requirements (including hospital, department, and job-specific competencies), including Back School, TB testing, Healthstream, and other departmental educational expectations.

        Yes   No

If "no," employee will receive a 1% reduction in their overall percentage salary adjustment.

LICENSURE/CERTIFICATION
Was documentation of required licensures and certifications turned in within specified timeframe?

        Yes   No   Not Applicable

If "no," employee will receive a 1% reduction in their overall percentage salary adjustment.

PERFORMANCE DEFICIENCY
Is there a Performance Deficiency that prevents this Employee from fulfilling his or her assigned duties?

        Yes   No

FIGURE 10.1
PMC Performance
Appraisal Form
Example: CFO's
Annual Review
(continued)

*If "yes," complete and attach a **Performance Improvement Plan**. This should be specific enough to give the employee constructive guidance on how to improve and how the employee can be successful in meeting expectations. Define a specific timeline for follow-up and re-evaluation of progress.*
Please note: employee will not be eligible for a salary adjustment until successful resolution of identified issues.

ADDITIONAL MANAGER COMMENTS:

EMPLOYEE COMMENTS:

Total Weighted Score	To compute the Weighted Score, please right click on the formula and select 'update field'.	0.00

An important part of the performance evaluation is a face-to-face meeting between the manager and the employee to discuss the evaluation. The manager should establish a meeting atmosphere that allows for interaction between the manager and the employee. This makes the employee a participant in the process and enables him to discuss his accomplishments over the past year, the challenges he faced, and the objectives and goals he anticipates. The manager's job is to deliver a performance appraisal that identifies strengths and weaknesses, shows the employee that he is valued (if this is indeed the case), and motivates him to improve performance. To do so, the manager should use a copy of the job description; pertinent reviews of the employee's performance from other staff members; a copy of the previous year's review, including the goals stated; and any other information about the specific employee's performance for the time period under review.

Another option is the **360 evaluation.** These reviews offer evaluation from the employees' superiors, colleagues, and subordinates. Palmer and Loveland (2008) note that 360 reviews may yield a more accurate and valid assessment overall by providing the manager with information from many sources, thereby negating individual biases. The manager, however, needs to be mindful that some evaluations submitted in this process may not be objective. Furthermore, Palmer and Loveland (2008) note that group ratings are more legally defensible than individual ratings on some issues, such as discrimination.

360 evaluation
A review process in which the supervisor, the employee, and staff members who work for the employee assess the work behavior and efforts of an employee.

10.3 TERMINATION CONSIDERATIONS

Along with recognizing, developing, and promoting talented employees, managers also shoulder the responsibility of firing employees. An employee who has consistently failed to meet expectations, failed to perform according to corrective plans, or engaged in an offense that warrants it may be subject to termination. If the manager has the facts and documentation to support such a decision and has followed the protocol for working with the employee to correct the poor performance, she should not wait for the annual formal performance evaluation (Thompson 2007). Observation, documentation, corrective plan action development with the employee, and follow-up should all be part of the process for the manager, the poorly performing employee, and an HR representative. The exception to this protocol is any behavior that warrants immediate dismissal (e.g., a hospital employee firing a weapon at the hospital).

Bucking (2008) offers ten steps to follow when an employee's performance may warrant termination.

1. **Know the facts.** Speak to all parties involved and listen to the information they share. In the case study, Dr. Daunt first met with Roberta, and she will meet with Dr. Fox to gather as much information as possible.

2. **Review the documents.** The supervisor should review the file of the employee in question to determine whether the employee's past reviews have consistently been poor, average, or outstanding. This review could indicate whether the incident is an anomaly or a reflection of consistent underperformance. A review of other employees' files allows the supervisor to note whether similar behaviors have occurred with other employees and to ascertain whether employees are being treated fairly. Dr. Daunt reviewed Dr. Fox's file and noted that his past reviews had been excellent.

3. **Create new documents.** Ensure that documentation presents an honest and direct record of the events. Dr. Daunt should keep a written summary of her meeting with Roberta, and she should continue to keeps notes regarding her future encounters with Dr. Fox and the HR and legal offices.

4. **Be aware of the electronic scourge.** Bucking (2008) advises supervisors that electronic records are not informal communications that disappear. Treat electronic communications as though they were formal writings.

5. **Tell the truth.** Be honest with the employee and other pertinent parties. It is not easy to let someone go from his employment. Be honest with the person being fired.

6. **Don't be gratuitously cruel.** There is no need for a person who is being fired to be treated in a cruel manner. If the decision has been made to terminate employment, then the manager should do so without engaging in a debate or argument with the employee.

7. **Conduct the termination respectfully.** Be polite and conduct the termination meeting without an audience. There is no need to fire someone in front of other employees. If possible, an employee should not be fired on a date that is special to her. For example, firing someone on her birthday should be avoided. Furthermore,

the day of the week the firing occurs is worthy of consideration. Some universities have a policy against firing employees on a Friday. The concern is that the employee may not be able to contact the HR office to ask questions about their employee rights until the following Monday, and the two-day wait may be too stressful for the terminated employee.

8. **Have backup.** If possible, the manager should have a witness present during the termination meeting. This witness, however, should not be a coworker (see #7). Rather, a representative from HR or another supervisor may be present.

9. **Pay all compensation due.**

10. **Think about other agreements or commitments.** If the employee has a company laptop, for example, the employee should be reminded to return it. Also, severance agreements may be addressed by an HR representative. Additionally, the HR representative could present a business card so the employee may make future contact if there are questions.

10.4 A Note on Sexual Harassment

The case study that introduced this chapter refers to actions that could be identified as **sexual harassment**. Managers need to know what to do if faced with such allegations.

Managers in healthcare settings should be aware of the potential consequences of staff members' behaviors. Sexual harassment is a form of sex discrimination that violates Title VII, the Civil Rights Act of 1964. The Equal Employment Opportunity Commission (**EEOC**) states that sexual harassment behavior includes conduct of a sexual nature that affects another's work performance or creates an intimidating, hostile, or offensive work environment. Any organization that employs 15 or more employees is subject to this law. During 2007, the EEOC resolved over 11,500 sexual harassment charges in the United States. The persons who made the charges and other aggrieved parties received $49.9 million in monetary benefits (See the EEOC Statistics at www.eeoc.gov for more information). Sexual harassment is not only illegal, but it can also cost an organization money that could be put to better use.

The following circumstances apply to sexual harassment:

1. The victim as well as the harasser may be a woman or a man. The victim does not have to be of the opposite sex.

2. The harasser can be the victim's supervisor, an agent of the employer, a supervisor in another area, a coworker, or a non-employee.

Sexual harassment
The illegal practice of unwelcome sexual behavior in the workplace.

EEOC
The Equal Employment Opportunity Commission, the U.S. government agency that enforces federal employment discrimination laws.

3. The victim does not have to be the person harassed but could be anyone affected by the offensive conduct.

4. Unlawful sexual harassment may occur without economic injury to or discharge of the victim.

5. The harasser's conduct must be unwelcome.

(Equal Employment Opportunity Commission 2008)

In the case study, Dr. Daunt's conference call is an important first step in addressing the situation. The incident appears to be one of sexual harassment. Roberta said the slide pictures were unwelcome and offensive. Further, the stomachaches she mentions to Dr. Daunt might indicate that Dr. Fox's actions are creating an intimidating and hostile classroom environment. The conversation with the university legal representative would confirm that the incident may indeed be sexual harassment and outline the appropriate next steps to be taken.

The EEOC recommends that organizations such as Medical University in the case study have a formal, written policy for employees regarding sexual harassment. The EEOC also encourages training employees in what sexual harassment is, what to do if they suspect sexual harassment, and what the effective complaint or grievance process is to address sexual harassment. Moreover, the organization should communicate the disciplinary options for any persons found to have engaged in sexual harassment. In each case, the scope and severity of the action would influence what disciplinary options are selected. Corrective actions could include reprimand, suspension, demotion, or dismissal.

DISCUSSION QUESTIONS

➤ What would you have recommended that the hiring team ask Dr. Fox during his interview to assess his level of professionalism? Keep in mind the questions that are and are not legally allowed during an interview.

➤ What should happen to Dr. Fox regarding his performance evaluation? Would a 360 evaluation be appropriate given the circumstances?

➤ Offer suggestions for a manager who is dealing with a sexual harassment allegation. Whom should the manager contact, and what should the manager discuss with the employee who has made the charge?

EXERCISE 10.1   WE ARE THE RECRUITERS

At St. Al's Hospital, recruitment and retention of qualified pharmacists was identified as an area that required attention. Teri Hill, a pharmacy supervisor, was called to a meeting by Peter Beachboard, the HR director for St. Al's. The purpose of the meeting was to outline, one on one, the hospital's new recruitment strategy for pharmacists. Teri didn't think the meeting would last long, as the hospital's hiring process for pharmacists had never really involved her. The HR department had always sent her approved pharmacy hires. She had only met with candidates as a formality.

However, when Peter stated that one significant change in the new policy was that Teri would now interview each job applicant, Teri realized that she had a lot to learn, and that this meeting was going to take longer than she'd thought. The HR department's new policy was that it would continue to screen applicants, and then it would send those applicants to Teri. She would be in charge of the hiring process after the initial screening. HR recommended that she rank applicants on a scale from 1 to 5 (with 1 as the best choice and 5 as the last choice).

Teri realized that this change would have an immediate effect, as she currently had three openings in the pharmacy.

➤ How should Teri prepare for her new hiring responsibilities?

➤ What questions should she include in the job interviews?

➤ What should she make sure the candidates know about her pharmacy department that would help them decide whether to accept a position there?

EXERCISE 10.2   IDENTIFYING SEXUAL HARASSMENT

JinMing Sue was hired to work as an HR representative at Medical University in Oklahoma. During his employee orientation, Harvin Fairchild, a HR senior benefits counselor, asked JinMing to review the EEOC sexual harassment guidelines.

Harvin said, "JinMing, welcome to the HR office. I am so glad you are working with us now. One of your responsibilities will be to serve as the EEOC liaison. As part of your orientation, please read the following cases and decide what issue(s) should be addressed and what decisions you would make in each case. When you are through, we'll go over the examples and talk about them. Oh, I am so glad that I don't have to do this anymore! Welcome aboard."

JinMing opened the case book and began to read.

Case 1: Maintenance Matters

Bill and Nils have worked together as groundskeepers at Medical University for over 20 years and are highly respected. They designed and planted a prayer garden for families of patients, complete with strategically placed benches where family members can sit and partake of the natural beauty during a potentially stressful time. The landscaping of Medical University's campus has often received praise, thanks to the gardening expertise Bill and Nils have brought to the job. If the nurses knew of a patient who had not had any visitors, they let one of the groundskeepers know. The patient would receive a bouquet of freshly cut flowers from the grounds to brighten her or his hospital room.

Several months ago, Florence Brighton was hired as an additional groundskeeper. It quickly became obvious that Bill and Nils did not approve of Florence. They told other people in the department, "Florence can't do the work and was only hired because she is a woman." The two of them conducted a campaign emphasizing Florence's shortcomings, got into arguments with her, and urged the nurses to complain about her to their boss, Hane Hightower.

After several weeks of this behavior, Bill and Nils requested a meeting with Hane. At the meeting, they contended that Florence was not carrying her fair share of the workload, and they resented having to do her work. They said that if Florence didn't leave, they would.

Case 2: The IT Training

Betty Summerton is the supervisor of Medical University's X-ray department. Sean Hartzog is a single male X-ray technologist. The university has purchased a new piece of X-ray equipment that requires intensive IT training. Betty has asked Sean to be the team leader for the technologists regarding the equipment. Sean is smart and good with one-on-one communication. He would have made an excellent teacher. Everyone knows that once he is trained, the other technologists will become proficient with the machine in no time. Sean will make sure the technologists are well trained on the new machine before he allows them to work with it. The IT trainer is Cindy Barton, and she has met with Sean on two occasions to discuss the machine. Betty has learned that Cindy has asked Sean out on a date, and that Sean has accepted.

Case 3: Physical Therapy Squared

Danielle Thompson is a physical therapist who is efficient, good natured, and a compassionate caregiver. She has been working at Medical University for five months. Danielle has come to see Sharon, an HR staff member. She tells Sharon that her supervisor, Ken, began making odd comments to her when they were alone within a month of Danielle's first day at the hospital. Then, he put his arm over her shoulder when they were working with a patient.

He patted her rear. This has happened three times. Each time, Danielle told Ken to stop and not do it again. But each time, Ken just laughed it off and told Danielle that she was too reserved. The day before, Ken had reminded Danielle that her six-month probationary review was coming up. "He told me I needed to get a good review from him, and then he patted my rear again!" Danielle took a journal from her lab coat pocket. "Here," she said as she gave the journal to Sharon. "It is all in there. Will you help me, please?"

➤ JinMing reviewed the cases and wrote a paragraph for each that addressed what he thought was the problem, options to help provide solutions, and, with reference to the options, his recommendations for addressing the problem. If you were JinMing, what would you have written?

    (1) Identify the problem for each case.

    (2) Offer a list of options that might address the problem.

    (3) Recommend a solution to the problem you identified.

CHAPTER 11

MANAGING CONFLICT

Xi Chang has been the supervisor of the local health department's home health unit, where she oversees 12 home health nurses, for three years. Her unit's performance is slightly but consistently higher than the health department's other units and divisions.

The health department hired a new director about six months ago. The previous director had always praised Xi for her high-performing unit and for her nurses' individual and professional approach to high-quality home care. The new director, it seems to Xi, is more focused on policy enforcement, financials, and the bottom line than on quality care and professionalism.

Recently, the director called Xi into his office to discuss her nurses' work and attitudes. The director is upset by the fact that immediately after leaving the main office in the morning, Xi's nurses congregate at a local coffee shop. The director made it very clear that this "socializing during business hours" must end. In addition, the director is disturbed that so many health department vehicles are seen parked in front of the coffee shop, which he thinks gives the health department a poor public image.

When Xi talked to her nurses about this, they admitted to some chitchat, but said they mostly use the time at the coffee shop to keep each other updated on clients, consult with each other on tough cases, and discuss care plans. Xi knows that their drive to provide the best quality care is keen and strongly collegial. In addition, the nurses view themselves as independent health providers who operate, for the most part, independently of the office and of the health department's other personnel. They did, however, offer to park their health department vehicles in the back of the coffee shop so they wouldn't be so obvious from the street.

Xi told the director that she believes that her nurses' informal conversations over morning coffee are key to her unit's high quality and continued high performance. The nurses are engaging in professional conversation, education, and consultation, which benefit the health department and its clients and should be not only allowed to continue, but supported and encouraged.

The director was not at all impressed. He sees no proof that these "coffee klatches" have any impact on care or quality. In addition, health department employees are only allowed two ten-minute breaks and one thirty-minute lunch period every day. This habit of taking morning coffee is simply a waste of time and of the health department's money. Xi needs to stop making excuses for them and start getting them to do their jobs.

Xi had hoped her explanation of the nurses' behavior would convince the director, but it has become clear that he is set in his opinion. Xi is offended by the director's negative attitude about her and about her nurses. Clearly, she and the director have very different ideas about how to run a home health service.

After studying this chapter, you will be able to

➤ answer the question of whether conflict is good or bad in organizations,

➤ delineate five styles and three dimensions of conflict, and

➤ discuss the effectiveness of a situational approach to conflict.

Relationship conflict

Tension, animosity, and annoyance unrelated to the specific situation and interpersonal in nature.

Task conflict

Disagreement about tasks, goals, methods, or desired outcomes.

11.1 CONFLICT IS EVERYWHERE

No matter how hard you try, you cannot completely avoid conflict. It is everywhere: at home, in the government, in your community, and at work. While conflict may be unpleasant, it is not always bad. It can be a positive force in organizations. Conflict fuels creativity and innovation (Whitworth 2005), maintains stimulation and activation, contributes to adaptation and innovation (Callanan and Perri 2006), is a source of feedback (Miles 1980), and can call attention to problem areas, thereby leading to a search for solutions and improvements (Amason 1996).

Still, conflict is something most of us avoid when possible. It is stressful and time-consuming. It can be perceived as destructive, a hindrance to performance, disruptive to teamwork, irrelevant to tasks, and harmful to relationships among coworkers (DeDreu and Weingart 2003; Chou and Yeh 2007).

Whether conflict is good or evil, it is bound to happen in organizations, and managers spend a significant amount of their time dealing with it. It is important to understand conflict and your instincts in dealing with it, and to have a framework for the better management of conflicts at work.

There are two primary sources of conflict in the workplace: relationship and task. **Relationship conflict** refers to "tension, animosity, and annoyance" among coworkers; it is often unrelated to work and is interpersonal in nature. **Task conflict** is disagreement among coworkers about the tasks being performed (Chou and Yeh 2007, 1037). Aspects of task conflict include disagreements regarding goals and competition or dependencies among coworkers or departments (Rue and Byars 2001). Task conflict in healthcare, as in Xi's story above, often centers on differences in approaches to work, philosophies of care, or priorities and desired outcomes. Task and relationship conflict are easily intertwined: When working with a coworker whom one doesn't like, it is often hard to agree on what needs to be done and how to accomplish it. Conversely, when one disagrees with a coworker about a task or desired goal, it is easy to see annoying habits and negative characteristics in that coworker.

11.2 FIVE CONFLICT MANAGEMENT STYLES

Regardless of the source of conflict, the options for responding to conflict can be categorized into five general styles (Chou and Yeh 2007; Callanan and Perri 2006). The names of the five styles vary, but they are characterized by depth of concern for one's stance in the conflict and for the other party's stance.

1. The **dominating style** has high concern for self and low concern for others. Dominating refers to demanding and imposing one's will on others with little or no concern about the impact on the other party.

2. The **accommodating style** demonstrates low concern for one's own position in the conflict and high concern for those of others. One example of accommodating is a situation in which you have no strong feelings one way or the other, but because the situation is important to the other party, you simply go along with the other party's wishes. Or it could be a situation in which you do not wish to assert yourself, even though you do care about the conflict situation, and you simply submit to the other party's wishes.

3. The **avoidance** orientation has low concern for self and low concern for others, and often presents itself as withdrawal or lack of cooperation. One example of this style is when the conflict is of so little importance to you, and you have so little concern about the other party, that you choose to ignore it. Avoidance, however, can be more malicious than just ignoring a problem; it can be passive-aggressive and highly uncooperative. It can be an attempt to control others not by what you do, but by what you don't do.

4. **Compromising** demonstrates a reasonable level of concern for self and for others. This orientation is concerned about keeping both sides equal and will attempt to match concessions, make conditional promises or threats, and actively search for the middle ground. The goal in compromising is to ensure that one side doesn't give in more than the other. Both sides do their part and give equally to resolve the conflict.

Dominating style
A conflict style involving high concern for self and low concern for others; demanding and imposing one's will on others with little or no concern about the impact on the other party.

Accommodating style
A conflict style involving low concern for one's own position and high concern for those of others.

Avoidance style
A conflict style involving low concern for self and low concern for others. This style often presents itself as withdrawal or lack of cooperation.

5.   The **problem-solving** style demonstrates high concern for self and high concern for others. It does more than search for the middle ground; it actively works toward finding the best possible outcome for all parties. It is assertive and cooperative.

Most managers have a particular, preferred style for responding to conflict. One might assume that the problem-solving orientation is always best. However, it is important to realize that "if all you have in your toolbox is a hammer, all issues start to look like nails" (Harris 2007). For example, you wouldn't use a collaborative, give-and-take approach with a young child playing with matches; you would simply say "no, don't do that" and take away the matches. Thus, an alternative way to think about handling conflict, the contingency view, "centers on the need for a flexible, rational approach whereby the choice of style or styles to handle conflict is contingent on a variety of situational factors.... The choice of conflict-handling style is a function of a complex set of personal, group, and organizational factors that dictate that one strategy is more 'situationally appropriate' than the other four" (Rahim 2002).

Conflict is almost always multidimensional (Jehn and Mannix 2001). When handling a conflict, you must take into account and balance the dimensions of **power**, **criticality**, and confrontation (Callanan and Perri 2006). Perhaps the most obvious of these dimensions in handling conflicts is power (Harris 2007). In the workplace, power can be based on status, rank, knowledge, level of education, reputation, or a combination of these and other factors. When the two parties have similar power, the compromising style, where each side gives equally, and the problem-solving style are often most effective.

In the case study, even though Xi has been with the health department much longer and has achieved consistently high outcomes using her approach, the director has more power. He has position and rank on his side, and, particularly if the health department is a strongly hierarchical organization, he may have the power to simply command Xi to follow his orders. The more power one has, the more one is able to use a conflict management style that is highly centered on self and unconcerned about the effect on others, such as the dominating style.

Another factor to consider when choosing a conflict management style is the criticality of the issue—the material effect upon the individuals and the time pressure involved in resolving the conflict. The more critical and urgent the issue is to the individual, the more assertive that individual's style should be. The less critical the issue is to the individual, the more cooperative and accommodating the individual can be. In Xi's situation, what are the stakes? What might happen if she chooses to disobey the director? Is the issue so critical to the director that he might fire her if she does not follow his orders? Is it so important to Xi that she is willing to risk her job or even her patients' health for it?

When considering the criticality of the issue, be certain that the issue is accurately defined. This is not as easy as it sounds, particularly when one is caught up in the emotion of a conflict. Is the central issue in Xi's story the nurses' coffee klatches, the health department's image to the public, the quality of care, the professional independence of the nurses, or the effective and efficient use of time and resources? If, for example, the main issue is the health department's public image, having the nurses park behind the coffee shop should resolve the conflict quickly and easily. If the issue is more complex, the stakes and criticality are higher, and both parties are more likely to choose more assertive conflict styles.

A final dimension of conflict is each party's willingness to engage in confrontation. Some people are naturally shy and reticent and will almost always choose accommodation or avoidance over a confrontation or argument. Others are outgoing and assertive and love to argue and force the issue. Our society often confuses **assertiveness** (positivity and self-confidence) with **aggressiveness** (hostility and combativeness). In the midst of a conflict, it is easy to cross the line from assertive into aggressive behavior. Some basic guidelines from Rue and Byars (2001, 323) follow to help those for whom assertive behavior is difficult to demonstrate greater confidence and to help those who are naturally assertive from crossing over into aggressiveness.

1. Don't try to place blame. This only polarizes the participants.

2. Don't surprise either party with confrontations for which they are not prepared.

3. Don't attack sensitive areas that have nothing to do with the conflict at hand.

4. Don't argue aimlessly.

5. Identify areas of mutual agreement.

6. Emphasize mutual benefits to both parties.

7. Don't jump to conclusions or solutions too quickly.

8. Encourage both sides to examine their own biases and feelings.

An entire chapter in this book is devoted to communication, but it bears repeating that accurate, clear communication is essential to conflict management. The eight points just stated are part of good communication techniques that can be used not only in business, but in your personal life as well.

11.3 SITUATIONAL CONFLICT MANAGEMENT

Conflict can be complex, emotional, and intense. It might seem natural to avoid conflict or to respond with anger, but smart managers learn early on to take a step back, clearly define the central issues, and think about the relative power of the parties, the criticality of the issue, and each party's willingness to confront the other. Once these contingent dimensions have been considered, a **situationally appropriate** style for handling the conflict can be chosen.

Assertiveness
Behavior that is positive and self-confident.

Aggressiveness
Behavior that is hostile and combative.

Situationally appropriate
In a conflict, taking into account the power and criticality of the issue and each party's willingness to confront the other.

Healthcare is hierarchical in its power structure and can hold the life and death of patients and clients in its hands. Before she meets again with her director, Xi needs to take into account these factors and her own willingness and comfort level in confronting him. Then she can decide what to do in this situation.

DISCUSSION QUESTIONS

➤ What do you think the central issue is in Xi's conflict with her director? Is this a relationship conflict, a task conflict, or both?

➤ Evaluate the dimensions of power, criticality, and confrontation in Xi's situation.

➤ Give an example of each of the five conflict management styles as they might play out in Xi's conflict with her director.

➤ Which is the most situationally appropriate style for Xi to use?

EXERCISE 11.1   TROUBLE IN BILLING

The billing office at Mt. Holyoke Regional Hospital is a converted inpatient room that has been divided into cubicles for the billing personnel. Wardlaw Martinez's and Harriet Lockwood's cubicles are located side by side. Wardlaw and Harriet have shared the small working space peacefully for over a year. However, Harriet has started a diet plan that encourages her to eat a lot of vegetables. Wardlaw is supportive of Harriet's effort to lose weight. It is important to her, and since she was diagnosed recently with type 2 diabetes, he knows that Harriet's success with losing weight is important to her overall health.

However, she constantly crunches raw carrots, raw celery, and just about any raw vegetable throughout the day. The *crunch, crunch, crunch* noise Harriet makes when she eats the raw vegetables is irritating to Wardlaw, and it is interrupting his work. The *crunch, crunch, crunch* has started again this morning, and it is only 9:00 a.m. Wardlaw sighs and stops working on billing. How can he do his work well with the *crunch, crunch, crunch* constantly coming at him? Wardlaw decides that he must confront Harriet now.

➤ What is the problem in this scenario?

➤ Indicate how the five conflict management styles may help or hinder conflict resolution between Wardlaw and Harriet.

➤ Which conflict management style(s) would you recommend that Wardlaw use when he confronts Harriet?

EXERCISE 11.2   THE APPOINTMENT

Laurie Schwartz hurried from the parking lot to the professor's office for her 4:00 p.m. meeting. Laurie is a full-time student, and as a certified nursing assistant (CNA), she works the afternoon shift (3:00 p.m. to 11:00 p.m.) at Rita May Heritage Nursing Home. Laurie likes her work with the residents of the nursing home. Most of the residents are appreciative of her care, and the few who are difficult are usually acting out because they are upset about issues not related to her or her work. Laurie has learned that patients are sometimes difficult because they are upset that their family members do not come to visit or because they are suffering from a health status such as a loss of memory and are unsure about their surroundings. Laurie knows that she has developed her patience because of her work with the residents. She takes great care to remain calm and reassuring to the residents as she takes care of their health needs.

In addition to her work at the nursing home, Laurie has returned to the university to earn her bachelor's degree in healthcare administration. She has not been doing well in her healthcare finance class. There is a lot of material, and Laurie knows that her math skills are not the best. She has been struggling to understand the concept of the time value of money. She made the appointment to see the professor earlier in the week via e-mail, and the professor had responded that 4:00 p.m. today was the best time for him to meet. She wanted to talk about the time value of money, and she was hopeful that the professor's answers to her questions would help her better understand the material. Her goal is to become a director of her own nursing home, and she is well aware that business acumen is important to her realizing her goal.

Laurie had to use comp time from work to make this appointment, and she arrived a few minutes before 4:00 p.m. to await the meeting. The professor is late, finally showing up after about 45 minutes. He tells her that there is a faculty meeting right now that he needs to attend. He asks if he and Laurie can meet another time.

➤ Identify the potential conflict in this scenario.

➤ How would you advise Laurie to respond?

➤ How would you advise Laurie to respond if the professor had missed more than one appointment with her?

CHAPTER 12

LEADERSHIP

ROSA'S IT VISION

Rosa Guiterez was the director of information technology (IT) at St. Nicholas Hospital, a community-owned hospital with 130 acute beds in a medium-sized Kansas town. Rosa had a degree in health information systems management and had started at St. Nick's four years before as a systems analyst. She had a natural aptitude for working with computers. In addition, she seemed to have the unusual ability to work easily with computer "techies," clinicians, and hospital managers. She steadily progressed up the ladder from analyst to team coordinator to IT systems manager. When the IT director position had opened up the year before, she had applied and had gotten the job.

St. Nick was like many U.S. hospitals in that its IT systems had been purchased and were being used without an overarching approach or plan. Departments purchased and used IT systems specific to their specialty areas with no consideration of their interoperability or their fit with the hospital's hardware platform. The result was that St. Nick's had small, stand-alone, proprietary IT systems that functioned quite well for their dedicated departments, but few actually inter-faced with each other. This **"best of breed"** approach to IT is common in hospitals. In this situation, IT departments must create interfaces and coordinate the stand-alone systems into the hospital network as well as possible.

While she acknowledged that best of breed was a legitimate approach to healthcare IT, Rosa had a different vision for St. Nick's systems. It would start with one electronic med-ical record system (EMR) to be used throughout the facility. The EMR would then be inte-grated into the hospital's admissions and financial systems. Eventually, all hospital departments and functions would share a common database with all systems being inter-operable and all departments and functions sharing and using the same information. This approach is often called an **enterprise resource planning (ERP) system**, and it integrates all computer functions of an organization into a unified system.

Rosa understands that many of the staff at St. Nick's see computers as a necessary evil—something they have to learn to use to get their work done, not tools that can help them achieve their goals. In addition, she knows that her starting point, the EMR, will set the tone for all future technology changes. Most clinicians still view the paper medical record as the gold standard, and it is going to be a challenge to help them see the advan-tages of the electronic version. Rosa's plan is to find one or two "champions" in each de-partment who will not only train their colleagues, but also demonstrate the advantages of EMR and spread their enthusiasm for it. She plans to create an IT steering committee and an IT task force, both of which will be composed of St. Nick's employees from a broad spec-trum of areas and disciplines, to help plan and support the implementation of the EMR and St. Nick's migration from the best of breed to the ERP approach. She knows that if the EMR implementation goes well, the entire organization will begin to respect her judgment about IT and trust her abilities to implement a unified IT system for St. Nick's.

Best of breed
An arrangement of IT systems that consists of many small, stand-alone, proprietary sys-tems that function well for their dedicated de-partments, but few of which actually inter-face with each other.

Enterprise resource planning (ERP) system
An overarching IT sys-tem in which all users share a common data-base and operating system, with all sys-tems being interopera-ble and all departments and functions sharing and using the same information.

After studying this chapter, you will be able to

➤ discuss leadership from an historical perspective,

➤ explain how leadership can be seen as a competency, and

➤ outline the exceptional leadership model, which is based on self-concept and built on the four cornerstones of

　　➤ self-awareness,

　　➤ compelling vision,

　　➤ a way with people, and

　　➤ a masterful style of execution.

12.1 HISTORICAL OVERVIEW OF LEADERSHIP

Leadership
The characteristic of guiding, directing, and assuming principal responsibility.

The Greek poet Euripides, who lived during the fifth century BC, said, "Ten good soldiers wisely led/Will beat a hundred without a head." **Leadership** is critical to almost any endeavor. But that raises the question: What is leadership? Is it something innate? Can it be taught? Can it be learned? Or is it simply something we know when we see?

　　Historically, leadership was often seen as something one was born into. Western kings ruled by divine right, and their progeny ruled after them. The idea that leaders are born, not made, survived well into the twentieth century with the assumption that business ownership would be passed from father to son. However, this view eventually gave way to the **Characteristic Leadership Model**—the idea that leaders possess specific characteristics, such as the following 17 qualities: ability to make decisions, energy, humor, sense of justice, determination, example, physical fitness, pride in command, loyalty, sense of duty, calmness in crisis, confidence, ability to accept responsibility, a human element, initiative, resolute courage, and enthusiasm (Adair 2005, 12). Clearly, not all leaders possess and demonstrate all 17 of these qualities. And many people who are not leaders share

Characteristic Leadership Model
A model that defines leadership as a collection of characteristics that all leaders share.

some or all of these qualities. So perhaps they are necessary but not sufficient to define leadership.

The next approach to leadership was the **Functions Leadership Model**. This approach holds that it is not so much the qualities that one possesses as the actions that one takes that define a leader. Peter Drucker, often called the father of management thought, proposed the following four components of a leader's job:

Functions Leadership Model

A model that defines leadership by the tasks and functions in which all leaders engage.

1. **Purpose**: the capacity to get the right things done, a clear sense of mission, and the application of talent and intelligence to the right things.

2. **Performance**: the consistent ability to produce quantitative and qualitative results over a long period of time in a variety of positions.

3. **Motivation**: A person motivates herself and others by having positive feelings about the job and possessing a sense of pride about the products and services of the corporation. The job is the avenue to self-development.

4. **Practice**: the job as a learning process. The key to effectiveness is practice, and as with any practice, ability to perform the job does not come automatically but can be acquired through constant learning. Effectiveness is a habit; that is, a complex of practices.

(Flaherty 1999, 281–4)

12.2 COMPETENCY APPROACH TO LEADERSHIP

Recent theory defines leadership as "a set of **competencies**, a set of professional and personal skills, knowledge, values, and traits that guide a leader's performance, behavior, interactions, and decisions" (Dye and Garman 2006, xiii). While one might argue that a leader is a leader is a leader, the high-stakes environment of healthcare presents a set of unique challenges. A number of leadership models specific to healthcare have evolved over the past decade. For example, the National Center for Healthcare Leadership's (NCHL) Leadership Competency Model, developed in 2004, consists of three domains and 26 behavioral and technical competencies. "The three domains—transformation, execution, people—capture the complexity and dynamic quality of the health leader's role" (National Center for Healthcare Leadership 2004).

Another example of a leadership model specific to healthcare is the Healthcare Causal Flow Leadership Model. This model is "a series of seven variables including three independent healthcare leadership variables, three patient moderator variables, and one dependent health outcome variable, linked in a causal flow" (Pelote and Route 2007). One of the healthcare leadership variables in this model is Leader Competence and Style, which encompasses 21 competencies grouped into the four categories of (1) Self

Competencies

Specific areas in which leaders must have the skills and abilities to function adequately and appropriately.

Management, (2) Power and Influence, (3) Logic and Reasoning, and (4) Helping and Caring.

While these two models certainly provide excellent descriptions of healthcare leadership, it is difficult to see how an understanding of them is going to help Rosa achieve her goal of an ERP IT system for St. Nick's. On the other hand, the Healthcare Leadership Alliance's (HLA) fifth competency of leadership, which lists "three areas that are central to effective leadership in health administration, particularly at higher levels: a compelling vision, energizing goals, and organizational" (Garman, Butler, and Brinkmeyer 2006, 360), seems a little too simple for Rosa's situation.

12.3 EXCEPTIONAL LEADERSHIP MODEL

Carroll and Edmondson (2002) suggest that "the mention of 'the leader' should not be taken to mean only the CEO or other executives. Leadership must be distributed broadly throughout the organization." In keeping with this, Dye and Garman's (2006) model for healthcare leadership is applicable to Rosa's achievement of the ERP. The Dye-Garman model consists of a foundation of a healthy self-concept, four cornerstones, and 16 related competencies and is depicted in Figure 12.1.

FIGURE 12.1

Dye and Garman's Leadership Model

The Foundation	Self-Concept			
The Cornerstones	Well-Cultivated Self-Awareness	Compelling Vision	Real Way with People	Masterful Style of Execution
The Competencies	Living by personal conviction	Being visionary	Listening like you mean it	Generating informal power
	Possessing emotional intelligence	Communicating vision	Giving feedback	Building consensus
		Earning loyalty and trust	Mentoring others	Making decisions
			Developing teams	Driving results
			Energizing staff	Stimulating creativity
				Cultivating adaptability

SOURCE: Reprinted with permission from Dye and Garman (2006).

FOUNDATION: SELF-CONCEPT

Self-concept is the foundation. This is your understanding of and comfort level with yourself. Most leadership materials focus on behaviors and competencies, but without a healthy and realistic sense of self, the competencies "will feel unnatural at best, and at worst will never be mastered....Leaders with appositive self-concept do not have to tear down others to bring up themselves. They rarely yell, scream, or curse, and they do not feel the need to play political games for their own gain. Their value systems engender a positive regard for others because they first have a high, but appropriate, regard for themselves" (Dye and Garman 2006, xxvii).

CORNERSTONE 1: WELL-CULTIVATED SELF-AWARENESS

The first cornerstone is well-cultivated self-awareness. Part of this is knowledge of one's own values and beliefs and comfort with living them. The other part is **emotional intelligence**. Emotional intelligence, sometimes called EQ, is "recognizing your own strengths and weaknesses, seeing the linkage between feelings and behaviors, managing impulsive feelings and distressing emotions, being attentive to emotional cues, showing sensitivity and respect for others, being an open communicator, and being able to handle conflict, difficult people, and tense situations effectively" (Dye and Garman 2006, 18).

Emotional intelligence (EQ)

The ability to recognize one's own strengths and weaknesses, see the linkage between feelings and behaviors, manage impulsive feelings and distressing emotions, be attentive to emotional cues, show sensitivity and respect for others, be an open communicator, and be able to handle conflict, difficult people, and tense situations effectively.

CORNERSTONE 2: COMPELLING VISION

The second cornerstone for healthcare leadership is compelling vision. Being **visionary** means creating clear and effective plans for the future based on a full understanding of the trends, opportunities, risks, and rewards. Rosa has a vision of what St. Nick's IT system should be and of the advantages the ERP approach will bring. Her problem is that few others will be able to really visualize an ERP and its benefits. Few people other than her IT specialists will have any grasp of the details, the expense, and the amount of planning and strategy that are needed to get there. IT has its own language laden with acronyms, nicknames, and technical terms. Healthcare then builds upon this with its own jargon, abbreviations, and complex processes. Clear and convincing communication in this situation is a must. Rosa's ability to work with computer specialists, managers, and clinicians will help her meet this challenge.

Rosa must help her colleagues understand the need and the rationale for the migration from best of breed to ERP. She needs to create a compelling story of where St. Nick's IT system is, where it should go, why it should go there, and how it is going to get there. She needs to tailor her communication to her audience; the hospital board of governors will have different questions and different concerns than the medical staff, the nurses, or the billing office. To build trust, confidence, and loyalty to her vision she must be prepared to connect her vision authentically to each of her stakeholders' values and goals.

Visionary

Having foresight, imagination, and the ability to form mental images of the future in a specific way.

CORNERSTONE 3: A REAL WAY WITH PEOPLE

The third cornerstone is having a real way with people. It sounds simple, but the most difficult factor in this cornerstone might be listening like you mean it. When you are the person with the information, the vision, and the passion, it is hard to sit and listen to other people's laundry lists of concerns and reasons your plan won't work. Listening is more than waiting for your turn to speak. Really effective listeners not only understand the other person's message, they also understand what is behind it. Many concerns or voices of dissent may be based on fear, lack of confidence, or discomfort with change. Perhaps more importantly, resistance often stems from a true concern that this is not what is best for the organization. Rosa has to realize that not everyone is as comfortable with, or as fluent in, technology as she and her staff are and that many people at St. Nick's might have legitimate concerns about this change in the hospital's approach to IT.

Rosa may already have a good feel for developing teams, mentoring, and energizing others. She plans to find "champions" in each department and train them in the new systems as they are brought on board. This is a tried-and-true "**train the trainer**" approach that is particularly well suited to healthcare IT changes (McGinnis et al. 2004). The creation of a steering committee and a task force composed of people from many areas and disciplines is an example of the entrepreneurial approach to IT governance that is recommended for healthcare organizations (Wiggins et al. 2006).

Train the trainer
The process of training one person or a small group of people, who then each train additional people, who then train more people, and so on.

CORNERSTONE 4: A MASTERFUL STYLE OF EXECUTION

The fourth cornerstone is a masterful style of execution. **Informal power** can be defined as the capacity to influence others without resorting to formal authority (Dye and Garman 2006, 132). Rosa's knowledge of computers and her way with people is a good start toward building informal power. The creation of committees and taskforces and her train-the-trainer approach will go a long way to building consensus and an open, participative team approach to decision making.

Healthcare organizations, particularly small rural facilities, tend to be traditional and cautious. Tight reimbursement and the large number of uninsured people in many rural areas result in hospitals having to watch every penny and to be excellent stewards of all their resources. IT systems are incredibly expensive, and the time and energy needed to implement, manage, and maintain them well is a huge expenditure for any organization, but perhaps more so for small, rural St. Nick's. Rosa's ability to drive results and stimulate creativity and adaptability will depend as much on her untested abilities as on the history and culture of St. Nick's and the hospital's ability to absorb IT expenses and tolerate change.

Informal power
The capacity to influence others without resorting to formal authority.

12.4 FINAL COMMENTS

Rosa's story is typical for many up-and-coming healthcare leaders. A young manager has observed the trends in her area of specialty and has a vision of where the organization should go. She has many of the leadership basics needed to implement this change, but she is untried in many ways. Using the Dye and Garman model, we can speculate on Rosa's strengths and weaknesses and the possible outcomes of her endeavors.

Leadership is a fine-tuned balance of skills, behavior, and art (Battistella et al. 2007). While no leadership model is perfect for every manager in every situation, they can serve as guides for healthcare managers. Healthcare is in great need of leaders. If not you, who?

DISCUSSION QUESTIONS

➤ Think about the Dye and Garman leadership model and pick three factors that you see as areas of strength for you. How did you develop these areas of strength?

➤ Thinking again about the Dye and Garman model, what are three areas that you see as your weaknesses? Create a three-point plan to strengthen each of these weaknesses.

➤ Pretend you are Rosa's boss. What areas would you suggest she learn more about? What specific skills would you help her to build?

EXERCISE 12.1   THE EFFICIENCY FACTOR

Hans Bellingham is the IT manager in a large family practice clinic in New York City. Most of the patients who come to the clinic are from low-income families, and Medicaid is the primary third-party payer for healthcare services. Consequently, reimbursement for services is low, and the staff must focus on cost containment to remain in business. Activities at the clinic are focused on increasing efficiencies so the clinic may remain financially viable. One recent effort has been to increase the number of patients a physician sees during the work day from 20 to 25.

To achieve this increase, Hans has implemented a strategic plan that includes the following:
1. decrease the no-show rate (the office assistant calls patients to remind them of appointment times);
2. rearrange the supply cabinet in the exam rooms to reduce physician effort to retrieve supplies and thus, individual visit length;
3. improve the workflow by reducing bottlenecks (move the copy machine from the hallway into a closet so the path in the hallway is open for easier movement); and

4. increase the number of exam rooms by reassigning the break room to serve as both a break room and conference room.

Hans was pleased that the staff had supported his ideas to increase efficiency, but to everyone's surprise, the increase in the number of patients per physician per day was not realized. Hans did not think that there was anything wrong with the plan. Other clinic managers that Hans knew had implemented similar plans with positive results. Hans thinks that perhaps some aspect of the plan is not working properly, but no one on the staff has been able to help identify what is not working.

This morning, Hans received a phone call from the clinic's billing officer. He had completed his accounting report for the quarter and was calling to express his concern. He told Hans that Medicaid was planning to reduce reimbursement again, and that the numbers "were not looking good."

➤ Review Hans's strategic plan, and determine what might not be working to help increase the number of patient visits per work day.

➤ Using your knowledge of Drucker's four leadership concepts, what would you recommend Hans do?

EXERCISE 12.2   EMOTIONAL INTELLIGENCE AND JOB PROMOTION

The committee for the HR director search had been working hard these past three months. Of the 21 applicants, five candidates had been interviewed by phone and two candidates had been brought to the Hot Springs, Arkansas, hospital campus for face-to-face interviews. The two finalists' references had been called, and the purpose of today's meeting was to decide which candidate should receive the job offer. The committee members reviewed the two finalists:

Evan Scott, an assistant HR director at a hospital in Oregon, was interested in the position because she had experience in the field and wanted to move back to her home state of Arkansas. Evan still had family in the Hot Springs area and wanted to raise her children there. Evan demonstrated great poise throughout the interview, listening to each committee member and answering their questions well. The committee members liked Evan's credentials and the way she had conducted himself. She exhibited self-assurance and confidence. The chair of the search committee reported that her references had been called, and all had said that Evan would be a good fit for the HR director position. A common statement made by the references was, "Evan is smart and just knows how to read people."

Catherine Curlington, an assistant HR director at a hospital in Texas, was interested in the position because she had experience in the field and was seeking an opportunity to serve as an HR director. Catherine answered all the interview questions well. She was smart, and her record showed that she had done a lot to help increase retention of the healthcare personnel at her hospital in Texas. The committee members respected Catherine's credentials and past performance, but were concerned about the way she had conducted herself during the interview. She had had an altercation with the waitress at the restaurant where they had had dinner, and the behavior seemed odd. The chair of the search committee reported that her references had been called, and all of them said that Catherine was great at achieving the CEO's goal of increased retention. A common statement made by the references was, "Catherine is smart and focused on what she wants."

➤ With reference to the tenets of emotional intelligence, whom do you think will receive the position?
➤ Why do you think Evan will or will not receive the position?
➤ Why do you think Catherine will or will not receive the position?

PART IV

TECHNICAL SKILLS FOR MANAGERS

CHAPTER 13

TIME MANAGEMENT

CASE STUDY   NOT ENOUGH HOURS IN THE DAY

Zoë Friedman, a manager of the hospice unit, peered between the stacks of papers on her desk into the hallway. It was nearly noon, and as co-workers walked past her office, Zoë wondered where they found the time to go to lunch. She couldn't remember the last time she had actually gone out for lunch. There was so much work on her desk, and her head was so full of details and deadlines that she almost always just grabbed something from a vending machine in the hospice employee lounge and quickly ate at her desk or skipped lunch altogether. Why did everyone else seem to have so much more time than she did?

Well, if she ever wanted to get caught up enough that she could actually go to lunch someday, she'd better buckle down right now and get on task. What was it she was working on? Oh yes, she was still working her way through a stack of papers and mail that had been dropped on her desk about 30 minutes earlier. Zoë mused about the amount of mail she got at work and at home. Here was an advertisement from a credit card company. She'd been thinking about changing her credit card to a different company, and this one looked interesting, but she just didn't know. She put it back on the stack of papers she intended to thoroughly sort through later.

Although she'd been putting if off for over a week, maybe this would be a good time to start creating an agenda for the hospice strategic planning meeting next Thursday…or was it Wednesday? She knew she had written it down in her notes from the last hospice management meeting, but where had she put those notes? Were they on her desk in one of her stacks? Maybe they were in her briefcase. Maybe it would be faster and easier to just call one of the other unit managers and see if one of them knew the exact date and time.

Just as Zoë was looking up the phone extension for one of the other unit managers, her best friend popped her head in the door and suggested they walk to the outpatient team leaders meeting together. Zoë gasped. "The team leaders meeting? Isn't that at 1:30?" Glancing at her watch, Zoë saw that it was already 1:25. She was supposed to present a report on the hospice's budget at this meeting, but she had only had the time to pull together a few preliminary numbers. Oh well, it would have to do. As she quickly pulled a stack of papers off her desk and stuffed them into her briefcase, Zoë asked herself for the tenth time that day, "Where has the time gone?"

LEARNING OBJECTIVES

After studying this chapter, you will be able to

➤ analyze how you use your time,

➤ plan how to better use your time, and

➤ use the provided tips and techniques to reduce stress and increase productivity in the work place.

13.1 ANALYZING YOUR TIME: WHERE DOES IT GO?

We have all heard a myriad of platitudes about time: A stitch in time saves nine; time waits for no one; time is of the essence; timing is everything; do not waste time for that is the stuff from which life is made; time is money. Why do some people seem so much better able to manage time than others? It almost seems as though those people simply have more time, yet everyone, including Zoë from the case study, has the exact same amount of time: 60 seconds in every minute, 60 minutes in every hour, and 24 hours in every day.

One way to approach time is to think of it as a limited resource, a tool you can learn to use and control. No one is completely **efficient**; everyone wastes some time. The key to time management, however, is to minimize time wasting and maximize productive time use. Books, tools, websites, and technologies are available to help you do just that, both at work and in your personal life. This chapter's approach to time management is not particularly theoretical, nor does it advocate a specific technique or product. It helps you analyze how you actually spend your working hours, helps you plan how to better spend your time, and then offers a number of techniques and tips to help you waste less time and use time more productively.

If you look at your schedule for the past few weeks, it is probably easy to see where you spent time in classes, scheduled meetings, and appointments. But where did the rest of the time go? Like Zoë, how often did you look up and see that it was later than you thought?

Efficient
Productive with minimum waste or effort.

Time inventory log
A tool that illustrates how time is used by briefly noting activities at regular intervals, perhaps each hour or half hour, during the work day.

One way to analyze your time at work is to prepare a **time inventory log** (Rue and Byars 2004). The log should briefly note how you are spending your time at regular intervals, perhaps each hour or half hour, during your work day. Choose a week that is typical of your working life, not a week when special tasks or events are planned for you or for your department. For example, part of one day of your log might read something like this:

Monday

9:30 phone call with Mary
10:00 e-mail
10:30 meeting with department heads
11:00 meeting
11:30 meeting
12:00 lunch break at desk reading reports
12:30 reading reports
1:00 preparing budget
1:30 talking with Bob

While this exercise may feel a bit tedious, it is well worth your while. Once you have a record of your time and tasks for the week, sort each entry into specific categories, such as scheduled meetings, telephone, e-mail, report writing, walk-ins, break times, planning and analysis, etc. Pay attention to trends and to which times of day you seem to be most productive or most unproductive. You might be surprised at how much time you are spending in some categories, and how little in others. After keeping a running tally of your time, how you spend your working hours should become clearer. The next question is, are you spending your time in the most productive ways?

13.2 Planning Your Days

Start by setting your goals and priorities. In the case study, Zoë is having one of those days where she is so busy that she is not getting anything done. She needs to start organizing and executing around priorities (Covey 1990). Working without daily goals and priorities is like driving without a map—you get nowhere fast. Identify what you need to accomplish, and plan your time accordingly. It is far too easy to lose hours of time tidying up your desk, sorting through mail, answering phone or e-mail messages, and dealing with unexpected visitors.

Open door management
Always working with your office door open to show that you are available to everyone all the time.

Clearly, part of being a manager is taking the time to talk with colleagues, coworkers, and employees about their work, tasks, issues, and concerns. Work would be a cold and boring place with no friendly talk or interactions. In our culture, we have a myth of the **"open door manager."** The idea of being available to everyone all the time is appealing, but not very practical. To become a skilled time manager, you must "develop the ability to say you are busy and that you can't talk right now to an unexpected walk-in, and let him know when you will be available to talk" (Credit Suisse Learning 2008). And if you have a door, it is okay to close it and work uninterrupted for part of the day.

But just what is it you should do when you close your door? Management tasks vary, not only in their immediate importance, but also in their long-term usefulness. This is called the "smaller-sooner" versus "larger-longer" **(SS-LL) dilemma** (Konig and Kleinmann 2007). This is a basic conflict between short-term costs and benefits and long-term, perhaps riskier, future payoffs. Research finds that people often prefer an SS outcome to an LL outcome (Rachlin, Raineri, and Cross 1991). **Effective** time managers need to find the right balance between both, while ignoring neither.

The first tool you need to spend your time productively is a calendar. Before leaving work each night, check your calendar for the next day's meetings and appointments to make certain that you are prepared for them, or that you have allocated the time to prepare for them in your next day's schedule. At the very least, this keeps meetings and deadlines from creeping up and surprising you and prevents the kind of shock Zoë felt when she realized that not only was she close to being late for her meeting, she had also failed to adequately prepare her budget report.

Next, create a running to-do list. Some managers pride themselves on keeping it all in their heads. However, most realize that as their work life becomes busier and their tasks become increasingly complex and time consuming, they need to keep a list of things to be done and their deadlines. A working to-do list includes daily, weekly, and perhaps monthly tasks. It includes tasks that may not be priorities now but will become priorities at a later date. Some people simply keep a running list on a pad of paper at their desks; some people use a calendar with enough room to write in tasks; some people use electronic or computer lists or calendar systems. None of these is inherently better than the others; the key is to find a system that keeps things from falling through the cracks and keeps you from having to call your colleagues for vital information like Zoë had to do.

Your to-do list should be reorganized and reprioritized regularly—perhaps daily, if necessary (Trunk 2008). Some people use a ranking system of "must do now," "important," "desirable to do," and "can wait" to prioritize their tasks. Some people simply number tasks or arrange them by deadline. There is no one perfect system; the best system is the one that works for you. "**Running a morning dash**" (Trapani 2006) is an example of prioritization in action. It involves spending an hour on the most important thing on your to-do list first thing each morning, even before checking your messages or e-mail. Running the dash ensures that your most important tasks get started and get at least one hour of undivided attention each day.

You may have heard the joke about the structured person who has to schedule "time to be spontaneous" in her or his weekly calendar. This might sound amusing, but work becomes tedious and stressful with no breaks or social interactions. While there may be days when you close your door, don't answer anyone's knock or the phone, and push straight

SS-LL dilemma
The basic conflict between short-term, more immediate costs and benefits and long-term, and perhaps riskier, future payoffs.

Effective
Having a definite or desired effect.

Running a morning dash
Spending an hour on the most important thing on your to-do list first thing each morning, even before checking your messages or e-mail.

through without a break for lunch, balancing work and your mental health is important. Zoë would feel better about work, and maybe be more productive, if she scheduled lunches and left some open times to engage in "office talk" with coworkers.

Finally, with the work stacked up on your desk, creating and working on your to-do list might feel like a waste of precious time, particularly at first. Shouldn't you just get to work instead of wasting time with list making? This is a good example of the SS-LL dilemma. The long-term advantages of taking time with your to-do list will almost always pay off in terms of long-run productivity and efficiency, so take the time.

13.3 WASTING TIME

The list of ways to waste time at work is endless. However, there are tips and techniques that seem to help most people manage their time more effectively and efficiently.

Like Zoë, many managers find themselves buried under a mountain of paper. One very practical tip for digging yourself out is to try to handle each piece of paper or e-mail only once (St. James 2001). Give each piece of paper or e-mail enough time and attention to absorb its message and then either (1) handle it right now, (2) file it in the appropriate folder so you can handle or use it later, (3) pass it on to someone else, or (4) simply throw it away or delete it. One has to wonder how many ads for credit cards Zoë has read and considered, then later reread and reconsidered as she continues to put them back on her stack of work to deal with later. Some managers swear by handling each paper and e-mail only once and actually go through their mail while standing up; it is too easy to waste time reading unimportant materials while sitting down. Standing up gives the task a feeling of urgency and gets a manager through a stack of papers or a backlog of e-mails quickly.

Also, become aware of your own internal clock. Are you particularly alert early in the day? Do you hit a mid-afternoon slump, or do you finally hit your stride after 2:00 p.m.? Try to schedule your most important and most difficult tasks for your best, most productive times. These might also be the best times to close your door if you can.

Manage your technology; don't let it manage you. Not every phone call or e-mail must be accessed immediately or dealt with that very minute. If technology interruptions are your downfall, try looking at your e-mail or answering your phone messages only at one or two specific times each day. As suggested above, try to handle each message only once, and fight the urge to click on every link that looks like it might be interesting.

What are your most tempting distractions? Is it your cell phone ringing, surfing the internet, getting a snack, or chatting with coworkers? These are part of work life, and you cannot avoid them all the time. However, as you become aware of which of them is most likely to lure you away from your work, plan in advance for ways to handle them. Strategies such as only chatting with colleagues at certain times of the day or bringing a snack from home can sometimes help you bypass your most tempting distractions.

Delegation is a vitally important skill to master. It is such an important facet of management that this book has devoted an entire chapter to it. Most people rise to the level of management because they are very good at what they do. It seems ironic that once they are managers, they need to delegate the very tasks and activities at which they excel and that got them into management in the first place. It often seems simpler and faster to do things yourself and ensure that tasks are done right and done well. However, this is another SS-LL dilemma. Investing the time now to train someone else to do a task will pay off later by giving you additional time to spend on other priorities. Finding and mentoring qualified workers to whom you can delegate is a vital management skill and can be an important factor in managing your time and continuing your success up the career ladder!

Delegation
Assigning tasks to others; the ability to get work done through others.

Nearly every time management book, website, or technology has a list of the most common time wasters (see for example, Rue and Byars 2004; Harvard Business School 2005; Credit Suisse Learning 2008; Gerard 2008). Our own list of time wasters includes the following:

- Telephone interruptions

- Visitors dropping in

- Reading and sending nonessential e-mail

- Lack of objectives or priorities

- Cluttered desk and disorganization

- Indecision and procrastination

- Perfectionism

- Inability to say no

Time management is about controlling two "eff" words (Blair 1992):

- Effective: having a definite or desired effect

- Efficient: productive with minimum waste or effort.

We sometimes think we can become more effective and more efficient by **multitasking**, or doing more than one thing at a time. Multitasking has been the time management tip for the past few decades. However attractive it might seem to be able to do many things at once, it may be better to focus on one task or one person at a time. Neurological research has shown that one unit of focused time is equal to four units of broken focus (Vaccaro 2003).

Multitasking
Doing more than one thing at a time.

"The absence of time management is characterized by last minute rushes and hours and days that seem to slip unproductively by" (Gerard 2008). Time management is not a genetic characteristic. We all know people who say that they just can't seem to get organized or that they just can't stop procrastinating or being late. With all due respect, they are wrong. It is hard to break old time-wasting habits and to learn new time-productive skills, but it is, again, an SS-LL issue. Invest the effort now to learn how to use time to your advantage. While you probably won't find all the time in the world, you should certainly find enough time to go to lunch. (And when you do, take Zoë with you.)

DISCUSSION QUESTIONS

➤ Zoë seems to have lost control of her time and of her day. List three time management techniques that would help her regain control and become more productive.

➤ List four time wasters that are causing Zoë to feel as if she has no control over her time. Then suggest ways to counteract each.

➤ Keep a time inventory log for a week and analyze how you spend your time. What are some ideas specific to you for making better use of your time?

EXERCISE 13.1   EFFECTIVE TIME MANAGEMENT AND ALICIA'S DAY—OXYMORON?

Alicia Benson entered the Cardio Planning Committee meeting late—as usual. It seemed Alicia was always arriving late to meetings. This one was focused on a presentation from the Utah Consultant Group (UCG). The hospital where Alicia worked as a health educator was in the process of expanding its cardiovascular services. UCG had been hired to present its architectural design for the new cardiovascular unit.

Alicia was asked to join the Cardio Planning Committee because she could represent the health educators' perspective on the expansion project and help keep communications open between the administration and the health education staff members. However, Alicia rarely spent enough time in a meeting to know what information to communicate back, and she was so busy apologizing for being late that she rarely contributed a health education perspective to the discussion.

Alicia settled in and examined the floor plan that UCG had presented. She did not see any space designated for community education regarding the influences of healthy lifestyle behavior on cardiovascular health. Why, she wondered, had UCG forgotten to include such an important aspect of cardiovascular care?

After the meeting concluded, Cal Hermans, the director of strategic planning, asked Alicia to come with him to his office. When they entered his office, he emptied a glass vase full of fresh flowers and water into the sink. He handed the empty vase to Alicia. Then he removed two pouches—one small and one large—from a desk drawer. The small pouch contained sand; the larger was filled with rocks.

Cal said, "Alicia, I want you to pour the sand into this vase."

Alicia felt this was a silly exercise and thought of the long list of things she still had to do today. However, since Cal was the director of strategic planning, she knew she needed to go along with his game, even if it was a waste of her time. Alicia poured the pouch of sand into the vase.

Then Cal said, "Okay, add the rocks." Alicia placed a few of the rocks in the vase, but could not add many because the sand was taking up too much of the space.

Cal took the vase from Alicia, removed the rocks, and emptied the sand back into its pouch. "Now," he said, "Put the rocks in the vase first."

Now Alicia was curious. What was Cal up to? She put the rocks into the vase.

"Okay, Alicia," Cal continued, "Now put in the sand." Alicia turned the pouch upside down and all of the sand flowed into the vase. Both the rocks and the sand fit inside.

Alicia looked at Cal and said, "I get it, Cal. Thanks."

➤ What did Alicia "get"? What was Cal's purpose for the sand and rocks demonstration?

➤ Why is it important to plan for the bigger projects first and then the smaller ones?

EXERCISE 13.2 WHERE DOES MATTHEW SPEND HIS TIME?

Matthew Morris reread a sentence in his management textbook: "One of the fundamental issues for a healthcare manager concerns where he or she should spend time." Matthew said to himself, "Ain't it the truth!"

Matthew was the IT manager at a community hospital. Much of his day was spent helping others learn how to use the electronic equipment, fixing mistakes people had made, and encouraging people to use the system and stop writing things down with pen and paper. The phone was always ringing; new e-mails came in constantly, and papers piled up on his desk. Matthew sighed, "I have to get things in order, and I have to do it now!"

Help Matthew organize his to-do list (see box) more efficiently. Using the information in this chapter, indicate what actions he should take and in what order he should address them for more effective time management.

Matthew's To-Do List

Goal Clarification
Current goals:
- Help the nurses learn how to complete the patient review electronic form.
- Negotiate computer maintenance contract with IT supplier.
- Develop presentation to teach new medical residents about electronic medical records. (The presentation is tomorrow at 8:00 am.)
- Help Katie in medical records figure out what happened to a patient's medical record.

Organize Workspace
Current tasks:
- Read paper mail.
- Answer e-mails. (Matthew has received 12 new emails in the last hour.)
- Answer voice mails. (The red light is blinking on his phone to indicate he has messages.)
- Clear clutter off desk.

CHAPTER 14

BUDGETING

BRIAN'S BUDGET

Brian Sage is the manager of the wellness department at Hope Community Hospital, a nonprofit hospital located on the South Carolina coast. Brian likes working at Hope and is interested in introducing new wellness programs. He has just met with Tony Benton, the chief financial officer (CFO), and he agrees that Tony's directives are right on target. The department's programs, while beneficial to patients and the community, were over budget last year. Tony is looking to Brian to develop wellness programs, but to do so within the budget. Tony has asked Brian to design a bottom-up budget that includes growth for new programs, and also considers profit-making activities.

Brian hopes he is up to the job. Tony is right—his department's expenses have been exceeding revenues. As a result, Brian knows he will have to ask for additional funds to start up any new programs. Furthermore, he knows that he and his department staff need to brainstorm about programs that might generate a profit to cover the educational programs that cost the hospital money.

Brian received his undergraduate degree in health education and joined the staff of Hope five years ago. His primary activities have been to offer exercise and diet classes to patients and community members. His excellent rapport with patients and his easygoing, friendly manner fit well with Hope. People like him.

While working at the center, Brian earned his MBA with an emphasis in health services administration online. When he received the degree six months ago, he was promoted to department supervisor. The administration had full confidence in Brian's ability as supervisor and his ability to grow the wellness department as a community benefit. The population was growing along the coast, and Hope wanted to be the hospital of choice for the new residents. The wellness department was designed to work with patients and members of the community. The wellness services would teach people about healthy lifestyles and market the hospital to the community.

In recent years, the cost of housing along the coast had increased dramatically, and retirement communities (housing that caters to people over the age of 55) offered financially well-off older people a beautiful, albeit expensive, place to live. As a result, the people who moved into the area are those who have accumulated personal wealth and are ready to enjoy their retirement years. They also are physically active and in relatively good health, and they lead healthy lifestyles. They are careful about their diet, do not smoke cigarettes, and do not abuse alcohol or drugs. Nonetheless, they are aged 65 years or older, and they have health conditions that reflect their age.

The Hope Community Hospital responded to this population by focusing on the development of its cardiovascular unit. Hope recently became one of the first echocardiography laboratories in the United States to be accredited by the Intersociety Commission for the Accreditation of Echocardiography. This recognition illustrates the high standards set by Hope in the detection and management of heart disease. Now, the hospital administration has established the goal of developing its wellness program to focus on their cardiovascular patients, and Brian has been given the task of proposing a budget that reflects this goal and, at the very least, generates enough revenue to cover its expenses.

After studying this chapter, you will be able to

➤ identify specific types of budgets,

➤ illustrate managers' use of budgets in the planning process, and

➤ explain the use of budgets as a control mechanism.

14.1 BUDGETING BASICS

As Brian develops the **budget**, he will keep in mind the following five points:

1. Who the organization is: What is the mission of the organization? Hope's mission is to consistently deliver compassionate, leading-edge healthcare to the people of coastal Carolina. The wellness department's mission is to provide the latest in health news and information, along with programs, community health events, and a fully equipped health and fitness center to promote healthy lifestyles in the community. Brian, with input from his staff, needs to determine what activities they want to support financially and how well these activities fit with the missions of the organization and the department.

2. What the organizational goals are: What are the future-directed tasks to be completed? Brian has been told that his goal is to develop the wellness department to focus on the cardiovascular population. New budget line items should be directly related to this organizational goal.

3. When the organization wants the goals accomplished: What is the timeline? Brian is developing the budget for the upcoming year.

Budget
A statement that indicates financial administration for a set period of time.

4. Where the organization wants the staff to focus: What is the priority of goals to be attained? Staff input regarding priority of services would help Brian determine what cash outlays he should request in the budget.

5. How the manager accomplishes (1) through (4) and stays within the budget.

Revenue
Income produced by a unit's actions.

Expense
Costs incurred by a unit's actions.

Profit
Total income or cash flow minus expenditures.

Excess of revenue over expenses
In a nonprofit organization, the remaining cash after revenues minus expenses.

Statement of operations
A statement that shows the revenues, expenses, and income of an organization.

Managers, however, can only do the who, what, where, when, and how if they know what they can and cannot afford to do. An understanding of their **revenues** and **expenses** allows managers to help their employees meet organizational goals and fulfill the organization's mission. Knowledge of budgets—what they are, what they are used for, and how to develop and defend them—is key for healthcare managers. If managers are well informed about the cost of running a department and they know what is being asked of their department, they are better able to deliver a plan of action that responds to the who, what, when, where, and how.

Brian has been charged to develop an annual operations budget that includes (1) anticipated revenue from future services and (2) expenses that reflect the activities necessary to provide those services. His budget is a written plan expressed in numbers (dollars and cents) that projects revenue (dollar amount earned from services provided) and expenses (resources needed to provide the services) for the upcoming year. Since Brian is responsible for adhering to the budget, he plays a significant role in its preparation and monitoring. Figure 14.1 illustrates the wellness department's operating budget from the previous year, which does not include the cardiovascular directive. The services provided by the department for health education and wellness did not generate enough revenue to cover expenses (the department incurred $10,400 more than it earned). Fortunately for Brian, the department's mission is defined as a community benefit and thus, his department does not need to generate a **profit**. However, Brian should determine how to at least meet his expenses and, if possible, to generate an **excess of revenues over expenses** (that is, make a profit).

As he prepares the budget, Brian should take into account factors that may change demand for the services of the wellness department. The growth of the retirement community along the beach area leads to an expected increase in demand for wellness programs for active seniors. Brian should remain realistic and project revenues and costs that are practical and are a good fit with the organization as a whole.

He also should consider the Hope Wellness Center's current economic status by referring to the center's **statement of operations** (see Figure 14.2). Overall, the statement of operations indicates that Hope's growth reflects the population growth along the coast and that Hope is in a good position to develop new projects that meet its mission to the community. Its patient revenue growth is reflected by its commitment to

FIGURE 14.1
Wellness Department Operating Budget 2008–2009

I. Revenue and Income

A. Inpatient Charges	$425,000
B. Outpatient Charges	150,000
C. Fitness Center Dues	25,000
D. Continuing Education Conference	12,000
E. Community Education Programs	-22,000
F. Foundation Monies	12,500
Total Revenue	*$602,500*

II. Expenses

Direct Expenses

Salaries	$400,000
Honorarium for Continued Education Conference	500
Equipment for Fitness Center	4,500
Materials and Supplies	62,000
Equipment Service Contracts	1,600
Advertisement/Public Relations	600
Total Direct Expenses	$469,200

Indirect Expenses

Employee Benefits (23%)	$92,000
Administration (Allocated 2%)	$28,000
Equipment Depreciation	$1,200
Equipment Maintenance and Repairs	$7,500
Custodial (Allocated 3%)	$15,000
Total Indirect Expenses	$143,700
Excess of Revenues over Expenses	($10,400)

the cardiovascular center initiative and the positive response from the community. From 2006 to 2008, net patient service revenue (gross patient service revenue minus contractual allowances minus charity discounts) and premium revenue earned from capitated contracts steadily increased because of service expansion. Other revenue (gift shop, cafeteria) and net assets (donor restricted to unrestricted in operations) have increased because of the growth in patient volume and visitors and the increased foundation operations to raise donations. Expenses increased as well to respond to the growth initiative.

FIGURE 14.2
Hope Community
Hospital Statement
of Operations (in
thousands)

Unrestricted Revenues, Gains, and Other Support

	2008	2007	2006
Revenue			
Net patient service revenue	$ 84,250	$ 77,650	$ 65,750
Premium revenue	$ 9,800	$ 8,700	$ 7,500
Other revenues	$ 8,700	$ 8,078	$ 6,700
Net assets released from restrictions for operations	$ 300		
Total revenues, gains, and other support	$ 103,050	$ 94,428	$ 79,950
Expenses			
Salaries and benefits	$ 54,490	$ 49,750	$ 42,750
Medical supplies and drugs	$ 28,770	$ 25,650	$ 19,350
Insurance	$ 8,300	$ 8,150	$ 7,950
Depreciation	$ 4,600	$ 4,430	$ 3,750
Interest	$ 1,850	$ 1,900	$ 1,825
Provision for bad debts	$ 1,600	$ 1,400	$ 1,100
Other expenses	$ 2,750	$ 2,500	$ 2,450
Total Expenses	$102,360	$ 93,780	$ 79,175
Operating income	$ 690	$ 648	$775
Investment income	$ 3,800	$ 3,400	$ 2,500
Excess of revenues over expenses	$ 4,490	$ 4,048	$ 3,275

Incremental budgeting
Creating a financial statement that is increased or decreased according to previous expenditures for a set period of time.

14.2 THE BUDGETING PROCESS

Four different forms of budgeting are used for planning and control: incremental, rolling, activity-based, and zero-based. If Brian were to employ **incremental budgeting**, he would examine last year's operations budget and add or subtract a percentage, based on expenditures. Since he has been given the new growth directive, he would estimate what percentage budget increase the department would need to fulfill the organizational goal. An advantage to incremental budgeting is that it is time efficient; however, it does not allow for an evaluation of costs incurred.

Zero-based budgeting refers to building the department's budget starting from $0.00. The manager does not refer to last year's budget as in incremental budgeting. Rather, the process requires each budget item to be justified. If Brian were to use zero-based budgeting, he would, in essence, "forget" about last year and provide a detail of resources needed to accomplish the goals fully in the upcoming year.

Rolling budgeting refers to the development of an annual budget that is reviewed in a specified timeframe (monthly or quarterly) and updated. A benefit of this practice is that the budget is constantly revised to reflect recent activities; however, it is time consuming. If Brian were to employ rolling budgeting for his department, he would estimate revenue and costs for the upcoming year and reevaluate the budget at monthly or quarterly intervals.

Activity-based budgeting involves allocating costs to each activity performed on behalf of the patient. Thus, instead of a budget that has a line item based on the department's costs (such as salaries and supplies), the budget item reflects the performance inputs and the costs associated with each activity (such as costs incurred to deliver the cardio exercise classes). Thus, Brian could classify activities as primary or secondary and those that added value to the patient and community and those that did not. Then, he could determine on which activities the department should spend more or fewer resources.

14.3 DEFINING REVENUES AND COSTS

The focus of financial controls for managers in for-profit healthcare organizations is to generate **profits** for the stockholders or owners. In nonprofit healthcare organizations, the focus is to generate profits for reinvestment in the organization. Both foci rely on the management of revenues and expenses. As Hope is a nonprofit, Brian's budgeting process is not focused on growing profits; nonetheless, Hope must generate revenues and control costs to remain in business. The wellness department delivers community benefits through health-centered educational programs and fitness center activities. Hence, operating revenues are concentrated in inpatient and outpatient services, program fees, and fitness center dues. Other revenues include donation funds and the interest from the donations.

Brian also knows that it is important to classify the costs of doing business so he may understand where the profit is made and where costs may be controlled. Costs may be fixed or variable, direct or indirect. A **fixed cost** is a cost that does not vary according to use (such as number of patients). To elaborate, one of the programs that Brian and his staff are considering is having exercise trainers lead cardio exercise classes at the fitness center. It does not matter whether ten people or 50 people attend the cardio fitness class; Brian needs to allocate resources to pay for the trainer. So the trainer's salary for the class is a fixed cost. Brian also plans to give each person attending the cardio fitness class a personal package of heart-healthy items. How many packages he puts together depends on the number of people in the class. Hence, the personal heart-healthy package cost is a **variable cost**: It will change as the volume changes. If Brian has 12 people in the class, he needs to purchase supplies for 12 packages. If he has 20 people in the class, he needs to purchase supplies for 20 packages.

Direct costs are those that are associated with an activity. **Indirect costs** are those that are not associated with a specific activity. To determine whether costs are direct or indirect,

Zero-based budgeting
Creating a financial statement for a set period of time that requires each budget item to be justified according to the unit's goals.

Rolling budgeting
Creating a statement that indicates financial administration that is reviewed in a specified timeframe (monthly or quarterly) and updated.

Activity-based budgeting
Creating a statement that focuses on the manager's allocating costs to each activity performed on behalf of the unit's responsibilities (such as patient care).

Fixed costs
Expenses that will be incurred regardless of volume.

Variable costs
Expenses that will change as the volume changes.

Direct costs

Expenses associated with a specific activity provided by a unit.

Indirect costs

Expenses that are not associated with a specific unit activity.

Brian may ask, "If this specific something did not exist, would the cost still exist?" For example, "If this exercise class did not exist, would the costs still exist?" If the answer is "yes," it is an indirect cost. If the answer is "no," the cost is direct. To illustrate, the cost of exercise mats is a direct, variable cost to the wellness department. The number needed varies according to the number of attendees, and the cost would not exist if the exercise center did not exist. To further illustrate, indirect costs (such as electricity needed for lights, air conditioning, etc.) are associated with the hospital as a whole and may be prorated by time allocated to specific departments. They are costs that cannot be specifically attributed to an individual project. See Table 14.1 for an illustration of costs that pertain to the wellness department.

Classifying costs associated with the wellness department allows Brian not only to know what is being spent and why, but also to explain and justify his budget. If he budgets for new equipment, he can explain why that particular equipment is needed to fulfill the goal. Projected usage and the acquisition of items may enhance patient care and attract new patients to the hospital.

Also, if Brian classifies costs as direct and fixed, indirect and fixed, direct and variable, and indirect and variable, he gains an understanding of what costs are allocated to his department, which helps him determine whether these allocations are fair. Rawls (2001) presents justice as fairness, and Brian can determine the fairness of the allocated costs only if he is aware of the actual versus allocated costs incurred to the department. Last year, his department was responsible for 3 percent of Hope's custodial care expenses. As he plans for the upcoming year's growth initiative, he may find that his department needs to assume responsibility for a larger allocation of the custodial care costs. This should be reflected in the proposed budget.

With the budget information and the program planning Brian and his staff will address, he will be well equipped to prepare, propose, and defend the budget for the wellness department. He will become knowledgeable about the cost of running a department; he will know what is being asked of the wellness department employees; and his department will be better able to deliver a plan of action that responds to the who, what, when, where, and how for Hope Community Hospital.

TABLE 14.1

Cost Classifications for Hope Wellness Department

	Direct	**Indirect**
Fixed	Brian's salary	Custodial contracted services (allocated portion)
Variable	Heart-healthy packages	Repairs of equipment in fitness center

DISCUSSION QUESTIONS

➤ With reference to the budget presented in Figure 14.1, construct an incremental budget for the wellness center. What percentage increase/decrease did you select? Defend your choice of percentage increase/decrease. Now, with reference to your budget, construct a rolling budget. What are the advantages of using an incremental budget for planning? What are the advantages of using a rolling budget?

➤ Offer three examples of direct and indirect costs in a healthcare facility. Why is it important to differentiate between the two?

➤ Refer to the following list and identify whether the cost is fixed or variable. If you were trying to contain costs, which set of costs would you try to reduce first? Why?
Costs of tongue depressors
Costs of occupational therapists' salaries for fiscal year 2008–2009
Costs of contracted-per-patient occupational therapists' salaries
Costs of rent for the wellness center's exercise site

EXERCISE 14.1   FAIR ALLOCATION?

Cassie Clemson, the clinic manager for the women's center, and Manuel Wentworth, the clinic manager for pediatrics, met with Tracey Farmer, the manager of radiology. Tracey had requested the meeting. The mammography unit, a division of radiology, was housed in the same building as the women's center and pediatrics. The women's center offices and examination and waiting rooms occupy about 40 percent of the building space. The offices and examination and waiting rooms in pediatrics are about the same size as those in the women's center, but pediatrics also has a play center for children, so it takes up about 45 percent of the building space. The mammography unit occupies the remaining 15 percent.

Tracey was preparing the mammography budget for fiscal year 2009–2010 and noticed that in previous years, rent, electricity, heat, and water costs had been split evenly among the three units. That meant that mammography, which only occupied 15 percent of the building, was paying one-third of the indirect costs.

She proposed to Cassie and Manuel that indirect costs should be allocated according to the square footage each department occupies.

What do you think Cassie and Manuel will say in response? Consider the hours of usage and number of clients as factors to consider when allocating costs.

What do you think is a fair allocation for the three units?

EXERCISE 14.2   DEVELOPING THE BUDGET FOR THE DIALYSIS CENTER

Gabe Richards, a dialysis center unit supervisor, reviewed his previous two years of budgeting for the center. He noted what had been budgeted and what had been expensed. Then he subtracted the difference. In some areas, he had budgeted more than he had expensed. In other areas, he had budgeted less than he had expensed. Look at Gabe's notes in Table 14.2. As he prepares the budget for the upcoming fiscal year, what factors should he consider?

Gabe had anticipated that he would be able to operate fully staffed from July 2007 through June 2008; however, the dialysis center was understaffed. How is this reflected in the budget?

Considering what has happened in the past two years and knowing that the goal is to have the center fully staffed, fill in the budget numbers for salaries, professional development, material and supplies, and equipment for July 2008 through June 2009. What increase, if any, would you propose for the center? Why did you propose what you proposed? Do you think you could defend your budget effectively?

TABLE 14.2
Budget Expenses for Dialysis Unit Staff Operations (Physicians Not Included)—Gabe's Notes

7/06–6/07

	Salaries	Professional Development	Materials and Supplies	Equipment Expensed	Total
Expensed	$ 1,233,041.57	$ 34,446.10	$ 241,001.66	$ 21,246.66	$ 1,529,735.99
Budgeted	$ 1,246,870.00	$ 66,528.00	$ 235,000.00	$ 21,000.00	$ 1,569,398.00
Difference	$ (13,828.43)	$(32,081.90)	$ 6,001.66	$ 246.66	$ (39,662.01)

7/07–6/08

	Salaries	Professional Development	Materials and Supplies	Equipment Expensed	Total
Expensed	$ 1,425,052.20	$ 58,800.00	$ 250,000.00	$ 23,000.00	$ 1,756,852.20
Budgeted	$ 1,534,548.00	$ 68,400.00	$ 248,000.00	$ 22,500.00	$ 1,873,448.00
Difference	$ (109,495.80)	$ (9,600.00)	$ 2,000.00	$ 500.00	$ (116,595.80)

	Projected 7/08–6/09				
	Salaries	*Professional Development*	*Materials and Supplies*	*Equipment Expensed*	*Total*
Expensed					
Budgeted					

TABLE 14.2
(Continued)
Budget Expenses
for Dialysis Unit
Staff Operations
(Physicians Not
Included)—Gabe's
Notes

CHAPTER 15

PROGRAM ASSESSMENT

AN UNWELCOME SURPRISE

If there was anything Jamal Bell didn't like, it was surprises at work—particularly surprises with bad news. How in the world had this happened? How could he possibly not have seen it coming?

Jamal had earned his bachelor's degree in health administration three years earlier, and after completing his one-year administrator-in-training (AIT) program for long-term care (LTC) administration, he had passed the nursing home administrator's exam in his state with flying colors. He had accepted the position of assistant administrator at West Wind Manor, a small, 20-bed skilled nursing facility (SNF), which was one of eleven facilities in the region owned by Healthy Elderly, Inc.

Jamal's immediate boss, West Wind's administrator, also had duties at the three other Healthy Elderly facilities in the county and was only at West Wind about one day each week. This meant that, as the administrator on site, Jamal was responsible for day-to-day operations and direct supervision of all the department heads and managers. Jamal had recognized early on that with such a broad span of control, he would have to rely heavily on the department heads and managers underneath him. Luckily, they had all been at West Wind longer than he, and they all seemed to know their areas well.

One of the things Jamal was proudest of was that everyone at West Wind genuinely liked him—managers, staff, and clients alike. He knew everyone by name and had an easy-going, friendly, open-door management style. He held monthly management meetings where each manager gave a verbal report of her area and was free to bring up any concerns or problems that had arisen. These meetings usually went smoothly, and Jamal and his management team often had time at the end of the meeting to discuss new ideas for programs and for the care provided at West Wind.

LTC facilities must meet a vast number of criteria to maintain Medicare and Medicaid eligibility. In the past, site visits by inspectors to ensure quality of care and compliance with regulations had been regularly scheduled, but they were now conducted on an unannounced, random basis. West Wind had not had a site visit in the two years Jamal had been there. That is, until the previous week, when the inspectors had simply shown up.

Jamal, of course, knew that his facility would eventually go through a site inspection, but he had not really been concerned, as things seemed to be running so well. West Wind's financials were strong, there was relatively low turnover among staff, and client complaints were few and far between. The facility was clean, the food was good, and the recreation events were well designed and well attended. So Jamal was shocked when the site visit team reported a large number of major and minor infractions. Jamal was given a short time in which to respond to the site team's report and to create a correction plan for each of the infractions.

If there was anything Jamal Bell didn't like, it was surprises at work—particularly surprises with bad news. How in the world had this happened? How could he possibly not have seen this coming?

LEARNING OBJECTIVES

After studying this chapter, you will be able to

➤ explain and apply a standard, three-step approach to assessment,

➤ describe a number of outcome evaluation models, and

➤ discuss root cause analysis and risk management.

15.1 QUALITY

Process
A procedure or progression of activities performed to attain a specific outcome.

In healthcare, the word "quality" often refers to the care provided to patients. However, patient care is not the only area where excellent quality is a goal. High-quality management **processes**, procedures, and techniques ensure that programs, departments, and organizations are run effectively and efficiently. Healthcare managers create the basis and the environment in which high-quality care can be provided.

Of the four fundamental management skills discussed in Chapter 2 (planning, organizing, leading, and controlling), controlling is likely the least understood. The word "**control**," in this context, does not mean ruling or being in command. Rather, it refers to methods of ensuring that things are done right and are on target. Jamal asks himself, "How could this have happened? How could I have not seen it coming?" The answer is that if there had been proper and adequate controls in place, and if Jamal had been systematically assessing them, he could, indeed, have seen it coming, and this disastrous site review might not have happened.

Control
Ensuring that work is done correctly and in an appropriate time-frame.

The standard **assessment** process looks quite simple on paper:

Assessment
The act of measuring, appraising, and evaluating.

1. Set standards.

2. Monitor.

3.   Take corrective action as needed.

(Rue and Byars 2001)

In healthcare, however, this simple-looking process can be quite complex, difficult to design, and even harder to implement.

15.2 SETTING STANDARDS

How does one know how good is actually good enough? How many mistakes are acceptable? In some industries, it is very clear. For example, few people would travel on an airline that reported that, on average, only 1 percent of its flights crashed. With many major airlines flying over 300 flights each day, this rate would indicate three plane crashes per day! And that is for only one airline! On the other hand, a student missing 1 percent of the answers on an exam would earn a grade of 99 percent, which by anyone's standards is an excellent grade. On the caregiving side of healthcare, setting **standards** is difficult. Each patient comes in with his own set of very individualized conditions, health levels, and preexisting conditions, some of which are known and some of which are unknown. In addition, each caregiver has her own set of skills and abilities. Given that the inputs (the patient and the provider) in any patient care procedure are so varied, how can standards for patient care **outcomes** ever be accurately set?

Standards
Customary, appropriate, and acceptable criteria.

Outcome
The end result, product, or conclusion to a process or event.

The answer is **benchmarking.** Benchmarking is the process of comparing one organization or situation to other similar organizations or situations using uniform measures. The financial world has long used a form of benchmarking to help investors decide which stocks or bonds to purchase: the stock reports printed daily in most newspapers. Anyone intending to purchase a stock or bond can compare one to another and thus make an informed decision. This type of performance comparison can also be applied to healthcare management.

Benchmarking
The process of comparing one organization or situation to similar organizations or situations using uniform measures.

For example, Jamal believes West Wind's financials are strong. Perhaps they are; perhaps they are not. What is Jamal's basis for this statement? Does he have specific, predetermined goals for West Wind's financial performance? On a more basic level, how would Jamal go about setting financial goals? To ensure that West Wind's financial performance is adequate, Jamal needs to compare West Wind to similar LTC facilities on a number of financial measures and set realistic standards. Jamal also thinks that West Wind is clean and that the food and recreational activities are good. But again, how does he know this? Jamal and his top management team need to take a long, hard look at each of the review team's areas of inspection and, using benchmarking, set reasonable and achievable standards for each area. Finally, the standards set should be shared and well communicated among the managers and staff. Everyone should know what is expected of him.

15.3 MONITORING

Once standards are set, there must be a process in place to ensure that they are being met. The long-established framework for monitoring in healthcare is the examination of **structure**, process, and outcomes (Donabedian 1966). Structure refers to the environment. Employees must be given the materials and tools they need to perform their duties. In healthcare this can mean the appropriate software to prepare a spreadsheet or adequate computing connectivity for billing Medicare and Medicaid. The refrigerators in the kitchen must keep foods that need refrigeration at a safe temperature. Buildings and physical plants must meet specific safety criteria, such as fire and building codes. It also means that employees must be properly trained and, if required, licensed, to perform their duties.

Ensuring adequate structure is necessary for quality performance, but it is not sufficient. Best practice processes have to be in place. Clinicians learn **best practices** in their own patient care disciplines. Accountants learn how to properly prepare budgets, income statements, balance sheets, and statements of cash flow. Human resources directors are taught legal and fair hiring and firing procedures. Best practices evolve; what was proper and adequate in the past may no longer be acceptable. Processes need to be up to date, well communicated, taught, reinforced, and upheld.

The final aspect of monitoring is the documentation, communication, and evaluation of outcomes. Information can be collected in a number of ways. For example, computerized inventory control systems can count and report the number of items, the time at which they were used, and those remaining in stock. Electronic monitors can record the number of people coming in and leaving the building. Supervisors can directly observe work as it is being done. Auditors can review and prepare reports. Utilization review committees can review medical records for best practices and appropriate care. Electronic medical record (EMR) systems can automatically record patient care and treatment notes and can enter items directly into patient statements of accounts. Important information about patient care and client satisfaction can be collected using interviews, surveys, and questionnaires.

Gathering the data is only part of the process. Deciding how to best present it is next. Dashboards are a quick, visual tool that can present information in an easily accessible way. Information reported in a **dashboard** format indicates whether the data meets the goal (green), are within a specified acceptable range outside of the goal (yellow), or fall to an unacceptable level (red).

Perhaps the most common way of presenting information is in a written report. Verbal reports, such as those presented in Jamal's monthly meetings, do not provide actual documentation and should be backed up with written reports. Spreadsheets and budget formats are additional ways to present information, but some people have difficulty reading and comprehending them. Finally, when reporting healthcare information and data, patient-specific information must be kept strictly confidential.

Structure

The environment and the set of conditions that exist. Structure is a necessary condition for quality to occur, but by itself it is insufficient to produce quality.

Best practices

Those actions, processes, and procedures used in a profession, discipline, or industry to achieve the highest outcomes.

Dashboard report

A report that uses color to visually indicate whether the data meets the goal (green), is within a specified acceptable range outside of the goal (yellow), or falls to an unacceptable level (red).

Any report, whether it is verbal, written, or in dashboard format, is just a collection of data. Outcomes need to be evaluated to be useful. Posavac and Carey (1997) present a number of evaluation models:

◆ *Traditional Evaluation*: The evaluator simply states her thoughts or ideas about the work done, with no comparisons to standards or best practices.

◆ *Industrial Inspection Model*: This is a one-time, "thumbs-up or thumbs-down" evaluation of the finished product that does not provide information on specific aspects of performance.

◆ *Black Box Evaluation*: The evaluator reviews the finished product and presents information on a number of key performance aspects of the product.

◆ *Objectives-Based Evaluation*: This method uses clearly stated goals and objectives and reports the degree to which these goals and objectives are achieved. It does not consider why the goals have or have not been met, or whether the goals were appropriate in the first place.

◆ *Goal-Free Evaluation*: This open-ended approach studies the inputs and outputs of a task or program, identifies positive and negative impacts, and then determines whether or not the outcomes have been compatible with the task or program's purpose.

◆ *Fiscal Analysis*: This method is an objective, bottom-line approach that determines financial viability, profit, and loss.

◆ *Expert Opinion*: Using specific measurable criteria as well as direct observation, an outside expert evaluates the product or services. The site review team of West Wind is an example of an expert opinion evaluation.

◆ *Improvement-Focused Evaluation*: Using quantitative and qualitative information, evaluators report discrepancies between what was observed and what was planned, projected, or needed, providing direction for improved outcomes.

Each of these methods has strengths and weaknesses. They can be used in combination to achieve a broad view of the evaluation subject. Many managers use only one or two methods of evaluation to cover all situations. However, the skilled manager determines which method is most appropriate in each situation and chooses the evaluation tool accordingly.

15.4 Taking Corrective Action as Needed

Jamal is required to produce a correction plan for each of the infractions listed in the site team's report. To do this, he must have a thorough understanding of the standard he is required to meet, a process by which to achieve that standard, a method for measuring and documenting the progress toward the standard, and a plan to correct any deviations from the standard once the process is in place. For some of the smaller infractions, the correction plan may be simply increasing the number or type of observations or implementing more appropriate monitoring and documentation systems. However, for the more serious infractions, Jamal needs to perform a **root cause analysis**—a basic tool of **risk management**—and create a correction plan to address the true source of the problem.

15.5 RISK MANAGEMENT

Healthcare managers need to understand risk management. The word "**risk**" means uncertainty, and managers must eliminate as much uncertainty, or risk, as possible. It is impossible to eliminate all risk, but the more certain the manager can be about all aspects of business performance, the lower the business's risk will be for adverse events. Having best practice systems, processes, and structures in place to ensure compliance with regulations and the law and to help decrease the likelihood of adverse events is an important facet of risk management. Adverse events tend to fall into one of three categories: human error, equipment failure, or systems failure, either alone or in some combination (McIlwain 2006).

Healthcare is human intense by definition, and when things go wrong, it is human nature to assign blame. However, root cause analysis, one of the most powerful tools of risk management, dissects the problem into its most basic segments in an attempt to discover the source. This is not a blame-seeking or blame-assigning exercise; the goal is to find out what is wrong and why and to fix it. An effective root cause analysis consists of data collection, investigation, determination, reporting of root causes, implementation of corrective actions, and monitoring for sustainability (Rooney and Vanden Heuvel 2004). McDonald and Leyhane (2005) offer the following six-step process for root cause analysis specific to healthcare:

1. Determine whether an immediate risk to patients or providers exists, and act accordingly.

2. Clearly define the role of leaders and facilitators, because effective analysis requires a multidisciplinary team made up of staff at all levels closest to the event and those with decision-making authority.

3. Determine the sequence of events, contributing conditions, and assumptions related to the critical event.

4. Analyze causal factors—those that, if eliminated, would have prevented the occurrence or reduced its severity.

5. Identify changes and develop action plans across disciplines. Implement changes through redesign or development of new systems and processes that improve the performance and reduce risk.

6. Present the recommended improvements to senior leaders for review and approval of implementation, including timelines, monitoring strategies, and reporting structures.

Clearly, Jamal and his team have serious work ahead of them. Creating adequate and appropriate correction plans for each of the site team's reported infractions will be time consuming and challenging. However, once appropriate controls and assessment mechanisms are designed and implemented, Jamal will no longer need to ask himself, "How in the world could this have happened?" And, hopefully, he will no longer be unpleasantly surprised at work.

DISCUSSION QUESTIONS

➤ Provide a healthcare management example of benchmarking. Where could the benchmarking information be found for your example?

➤ Assume that one of the infractions the site review team found at West Wind was noncompliance with fire safety standards—specifically, an insufficient number of fire extinguishers, inaccessible fire extinguishers, and insufficient testing of fire extinguishers. Propose a correction plan of standards, monitoring, and corrective action.

➤ The beginning of this chapter states that although the standard assessment process might look simple on paper, it is complex and often hard to implement in healthcare settings. What specific factors might make assessment more challenging in healthcare than in other industries?

EXERCISE 15.1   WHAT DISNEY CAN TEACH WALTER REED

The U.S. Army is paying Walt Disney, Inc., $800,000 in consultant fees to serve as a benchmark regarding its treatment of veterans. Walter Reed Army Medical Center has received unfavorable reviews from veterans frustrated by receiving the "runaround," not getting their questions answered, being constantly faced with an impersonal bureaucracy, and being cared for in a shabby, if not unhealthy, environment (Vogel 2008).

Walt Disney, Inc., will help Walter Reed Army Medical Center by sharing best practices regarding customer service. Walter Reed staff members hope that they can put the "care" back into "healthcare" for the veterans.

➤ What common ground do you think Disney shares with Walter Reed?

➤ How would you recommend that Walter Reed Army Medical Center evaluate the program's outcomes for the treatment of veterans?

EXERCISE 15.2   PATIENT SAFETY AND THE TOYOTA MODEL

Dr. Sunithi Narayani left the hospital board meeting in a huff. She was not happy with the vote the board had just taken. They had elected to pay for hospital leaders to travel to Japan to visit the Toyota manufacturing plants. "People are not cars," snorted Dr. Narayani. "This is ridiculous, and I have to go to Japan for this? My patients need me here."

The majority of the board members of California's Wellness and Optimal Health Clinic, located near the coast in Santa Barbara, had approved Clinic Manager Katie Springer's proposal that they travel to Japan to learn firsthand about Taiichi Ohno's Toyota Production System. The Toyota Production System focuses on actions that can eliminate waste and defects in car production. If a worker on the assembly line notices a defect, the entire line is stopped and the problem is addressed immediately. Katie thought that patient errors might be reduced if the clinic adapted a similar strategy. Any healthcare worker could stop a procedure if he or she noticed a problem that could bring about an error in patient care.

Furthermore, the timing of patient interactions could help reduce inefficiencies. Instead of waiting until the end of the day to go through each patient's chart and add information, a physician could write down comments immediately after seeing a patient. This would increase time efficiencies for the physician and potentially decrease errors in patient records.

Katie was looking forward to seeing the techniques board members might learn in Japan and bring back to California. She was hopeful that Dr. Narayani would understand the value these efficiency-producing measures could bring to patient care once she saw them firsthand.

➤ Assume you are Katie, and Dr. Narayani wants to discuss this trip with you. What do you say to influence the doctor to keep an open mind regarding the Toyota Production System and its application to healthcare?

➤ How does an effort such as this help with program assessment of the clinic? Consider best practices and evaluation methods in your answer.

➤ Think of two examples where patient error might be reduced if the clinic adopts aspects of the Toyota Production System.

CHAPTER 16

LEGAL ISSUES

THE LAWSUIT

Pat Wheeler was the new administrator of City Multispecialty Group (CMG), the largest physician group practice in the area. It was the end of her third week, and as she prepared to leave for the weekend, she congratulated herself on how easily she had stepped into the job.

Just then her assistant, Joy, buzzed her on the intercom to say that the group's attorney was on the phone asking to set up an appointment to discuss the lawsuit. "What lawsuit? I don't know anything about any lawsuits," Pat said.

Joy replied, "Well, should I give him an appointment?"

After a few seconds of thought, Pat said, "Sure, but don't make it until the middle of the week. I need to talk with Mark and Linda and see if they know anything about this."

Mark Winkel was CMG's former administrator. When Pat took over the position, Mark told her to call him anytime for help or advice. Linda Crane, MD, was the group's president and medical director.

First thing Monday morning, Pat called Mark and Linda and set up a meeting for that afternoon. When they arrived in Pat's office later that day, Pat asked them point blank whether they knew of any outstanding and ongoing legal issues for CMG. After a few seconds, Mark responded, "Oh, I bet I might know what this is about. Right before I left, I had to fire one of the nurses because we thought she was spilling information about patients. She was pretty steamed about being let go. Maybe she's suing us. Boy, I had the hardest time finding someone to replace her."

"Weren't there many applicants?" asked Pat. "I thought that when I interviewed, you said that staffing wasn't an issue for CMG."

"Well, yeah, there were plenty of applicants," Mark replied, "but you know, we have to be very careful about appearances here and I couldn't believe how many overweight, unattractive nurses I interviewed...and so many of them had such strong accents that I could barely understand them. Finally, Chris down in OB applied, and I hired her right away. She's worked out really well. Anyway, I didn't think any of this would actually come to a lawsuit."

Pat looked up from the notes she was taking. "Is there anything else?" she asked.

Mark said, "Well, let me think. I guess about a year ago, some folks were asking questions about how CMG was formed. You know, we merged the only two multispecialty clinics in the area. But I don't think that ever came to be anything. Oh, and there is always that rumor that some of the physicians in the group only refer patients to each other and to their own labs."

At this point, Linda interjected, "But no one has ever been able to prove that."

After an uncomfortable silence, Pat asked if there were any other legal concerns that they needed to talk about. "There aren't any malpractice suits, are there?" she asked.

"Nope, none that we know about," said Linda. With this, the meeting ended.

After Mark and Linda had left her office, Pat got up and closed her door. There had been no hint of any of this when she interviewed. Her appointment with CMG's attorney was the day after tomorrow. What should she do? How should she handle this?

LEARNING OBJECTIVES

After studying this chapter, you will be able to

➤ outline the broad and overarching legislation imposed by the government and

➤ discuss the legal duties and responsibilities shared among

- health organizations
- patients
- physicians, and
- employees.

16.1 HEALTHCARE AND THE LAW

It is imperative that healthcare managers understand their industry's complex legal environment. Healthcare managers face legal issues every day (but hopefully not as many in any one day as Pat is facing in the case study). Of course, all health professionals, managers, and organizations must obey the same laws as other businesses and citizens, such as tax law, contract law, and business law. However, the special circumstances of healthcare have resulted in additional, healthcare-specific laws and regulations. These laws and regulations are far too numerous to be discussed individually in this chapter. Therefore, without going into specifics or detailed discussion and analysis of individual laws, this chapter presents a general overview of health law, first looking at broad and overarching legislation imposed by the government and then examining the legal duties and responsibilities of health organizations, patients, physicians, and employees. Unless otherwise noted, the term *health organization* applies to any organization or facility that delivers healthcare, including, but not limited to, hospitals, LTC facilities, behavioral and mental health facilities, physician group practices, and clinics of any sort. The term *provider* applies to any and all caregivers.

16.2 FEDERAL LAW

For the most part, federal laws that affect health organizations and providers are intended to prevent fraud, abuse, corruption, and the waste of government monies. While government

Antitrust legislation
Laws established to prevent the formation of monopolies or other business structures that prevent free trade or attempt to restrain commerce.

Kickback
A form of bribery; the offering, giving, receiving, or soliciting of any item of value to influence the actions of another.

Bribe
A gift bestowed to influence the receiver's conduct.

Emergency Medical Treatment and Active Labor Law Act of 1986 (EMTALA)
Legislation created to address the perceived concern of "patient dumping"—the refusal to treat uninsured patients and to instead transfer them to charitable hospitals without having been seen or having gotten any care. EMTALA requires hospitals and their affiliated physicians to screen and to continue to treat emergency patients until they are stabilized or transferred.

funding for health organizations and providers comes from various sources, the federal laws discussed here have been primarily designed to protect the government's investments in the Medicare and Medicaid programs.

Antitrust legislation exists to ensure competition. The Sherman Antitrust Act of 1890 prevents restraint of trade and formation of monopolies, and the Federal Trade Commission Act of 1914 outlaws unfair competition and deceptive acts or practices. The Clayton Act of 1914 addresses contracting and exclusive dealing arrangements, and the Robinson-Patman Act of 1936 stops price discrimination. These antitrust acts were legislated many years ago and were not specifically directed at healthcare. However, they have become increasingly pertinent to healthcare. Recent decades have seen an unprecedented number of mergers, acquisitions, joint ventures, and contractual relationships among health organizations, providers, insurers, physician groups, and vendors. When CMG was formed by merging the only two multispecialty groups in the region, there could have been cause for antitrust concerns. However, because not all physicians in the area are members of CMG, and because other specialty-specific group practices still exist in the area, it is unlikely that CMG has monopoly power.

The Medicare Fraud and Abuse Amendments of 1977 and the Medicare and Medicaid Patient and Program Protection Act of 1987 are commonly known as Stark I and Stark II, and they include what is known as the Anti-Kickback Statute. A **kickback**, a form of bribery, is the "offering, giving, receiving, or soliciting of any item of value to influence the actions of the other person. The **bribe** is the gift bestowed to influence the receiver's conduct" (Garner 2004). In this case, it is an offer of payment in exchange for referrals. The Stark rulings also forbid organizations and providers from referring patients to themselves or to businesses in which they hold an ownership position (Hastings, Luce, and Wynstra 1995, 85). Anti-kickback laws were created to ensure free trade and the patient's free choice of provider. In addition, the regulation of referrals is meant to prevent the creation of feedback loops of referrals and services that benefit the organization or providers but may not be in the best interests of the patient. Dr. Crane's assertion that there has never been any proof of this at CMG implies that the group's referral patterns have been a matter of concern. Pat needs to find out whether there has been any previous action against CMG in regard to referrals, and if so, how it was resolved.

The last federal law to be discussed in this section is the **Emergency Medical Treatment and Active Labor Law Act of 1986 (EMTALA)** which applies most directly to hospitals. EMTALA was created to address the perceived concern of "patient dumping"— the refusal to treat uninsured patients, transferring them instead to charitable hospitals without them having been seen or having gotten care (Centers for Medicare & Medicaid Services 2007). Previously, common law in many states held physicians and health organizations under no obligation to treat any person seeking care. To prevent patient dumping, EMTALA requires hospitals and their affiliated physicians to screen and continue to treat emergency patients until they are stabilized or transferred (Healthlinks 2007).

16.3 HEALTHCARE ORGANIZATIONS AND PATIENTS

While EMTALA clarifies the hospital's duties to emergency patients, the hospital's obligation to treat in nonemergency situations is less clear. For example, a hospital may decline to provide care if it does not have adequate facilities or providers. In addition, a hospital may require that patients be admitted by an attending physician who is a member of the hospital's medical staff. On the other hand, Title VI of the Civil Rights Act of 1964, Section 504 of the Rehabilitation Act of 1973, and Title III of the Older American Amendments of 1975 provide hospital patients protection from discrimination. Finally, once a patient has been accepted and treated, a contract is implied—a hospital or provider may not simply stop treating that patient without risking **liability** for abandonment (Pozgar 1993, 84).

Health organizations and providers have the duty to maintain complete, accurate, and timely medical records for all treated patients. The medical record is more than just documentation of the care and treatment provided. Medical records are used to review the appropriateness of care, to provide information for billing, and as a data source for medical research. The medical record is in some sense a legal document, and it may be used as evidence in **malpractice** cases or other legal proceedings. Medical records must be confidential, secure, current, authenticated, legible, and complete (The Joint Commission 1995).

In addition to the obligation to maintain medical records, hospitals are responsible for keeping all patient-specific information safe and confidential. The **Health Insurance Portability and Accountability Act's (HIPAA) Privacy Rule** took effect in 2003. "The HIPAA Privacy Rule establishes a 'floor of safeguards' to protect confidentiality and privacy" (Wager, Lee, and Glaser 2005, 82) and was the first federal law to specifically identify **protected health information (PHI)**. PHI is information that

- relates to a person's physical or mental health, the provision of healthcare, or the payment for healthcare;

- identifies the person who is the subject of the information;

- is created or received by an entity subject to HIPAA; and

- is transmitted or maintained in any form (paper, electronic, or oral)

  (Wager, Lee, and Glaser 2005, 84–85).

Despite the need to protect PHI, health organizations and providers may be required to release information in certain circumstances. For example, federal law requires the reporting of certain incidents relating to the failure or malfunction of medical devices. In addition, some states require providers to report suspected cases of child abuse, elder abuse

Liability
Being in a position to likely incur an undesirable responsibility or obligation, usually monetary.

Malpractice
Injury or harm to a patient or customer directly caused by negligence, intentional tort, or breach of contract by a professional.

Health Insurance Portability and Accountability Act's (HIPAA) Privacy Rule
Part of the Health Insurance Portability and Accountability Act that establishes safeguards to protect confidentiality and privacy and specifically identifies protected health information.

Protected health information (PHI)
Information from which a specific person or patient can be identified and that relates to physical or mental health, the provision of healthcare, or the payment for healthcare.

or neglect, births, deaths, gunshot wounds, and some contagious, infectious, and occupational diseases (Hastings, Luce, and Wynstra 1995). Health providers may also release PHI for quality, utilization, and peer review; third-party payment; program evaluation; or medical research.

In the case study, Mark thinks the lawsuit might be about the nurse who was fired for breaching confidentiality. It is unclear whether she was actually divulging patient information or was simply suspected of it. If she was breaking confidentiality and if this is the subject of the lawsuit, this is a serious matter, and CMG could be at great risk. Even if this is not the matter of the lawsuit, Pat should review the circumstances of this nurse's release. In addition, Pat needs to review and, if necessary, revise CMG's policies and procedures on confidentiality.

16.4 Healthcare Organizations and Physicians

Hospitals are required to have an organized medical staff of physicians and other licensed providers who have privileges at that hospital and are authorized to treat patients in that facility. Because members of the medical staff are often not hospital employees, a mechanism is needed to ensure the quality of services and care within the organization. Health organizations need clear and enforceable criteria for medical staff membership. Since lawsuits are often directed at the provider and the organization, health organizations and their boards of directors need to demonstrate due diligence in allowing the privilege of practicing in their facilities. They too can be liable if they should have reasonably known that a medical staff member was not meeting the quality standards of care required.

Antitrust is another area to consider. Even when a hospital has clear criteria for appointing and maintaining its medical staff, physicians have challenged staff membership under antitrust laws—primarily the Sherman Act, which prohibits restraint of trade. Physicians in practice groups must also be aware of antitrust activities and are prohibited from acting together to:

- refuse to accept a proposed fee schedule from a payor;
- merge so all physicians in a specialty in a service area are in one group; or
- vote to refuse hospital privileges for a new physician if that means that physician will not be able to practice in the service area.

(Wenzel and Wenzel 2005, 199)

Based on these three criteria and the fact that there are a number of specialty-specific groups in the area, it is unlikely that CMG is guilty of forming a monopoly or causing restraint of trade in its service area.

16.5 PROVIDERS AND PATIENTS

Providers are generally under no legal obligation to accept or treat any individual unless they have entered into a contract for care with a managed care organization, a hospital, or another such entity. However, once a provider has accepted an individual as a patient, a contract for care is implied. Once the provider–patient relationship has been established, the provider must continue to provide care and fulfill her responsibilities to the patient until the relationship is legally terminated, or she may be held liable for abandonment.

Even if the provider–patient relationship exists, the provider must obtain the patient's consent before providing medical treatment, as patients have the right to refuse treatment. Obtaining **informed consent** from the patient is the duty of the provider. "Informed consent is a legal document in all 50 states. It is an agreement for a proposed medical treatment or non-treatment, or for a proposed invasive procedure. It requires physicians to disclose the benefits, risks, and alternatives to the proposed treatment, non-treatment, or procedure. It is the method by which fully informed, rational persons may be involved in choices about their health care" (Encyclopedia of Surgery 2007).

There are two criteria for informed consent. First, the information provided to the patient must meet the standard of the "reasonable provider"—the information that a reasonable provider in the same specialty would disclose under the same circumstances. The second criterion is the standard of the "reasonable patient"—the information that a reasonable patient in the same circumstances would want and need to know to make an informed decision regarding the proposed treatment (Encyclopedia of Surgery 2007). Failure of a provider to meet both criteria may constitute grounds for liability and perhaps illegal touching in the form of battery (American Medical Association 2007).

A final topic in the area of providers and patients is one with which most people are familiar, the issue of professional liability or malpractice. Malpractice cases can arise because of alleged negligence, intentional **tort**, or breach of contract (Showalter 2007, 39). A tort is an intentional wrong that results in injury; breach of contract is a category of tort. Negligence, the most common cause of professional liability actions, has four elements that must be proven: (1) that the provider had duty of due care, (2) that the provider breached that duty, (3) that the provider's breach of duty was the direct cause of the injury, and (4) that the injury resulted in damages to the patient (Showalter 2007, 39).

Linda's assertion that there are no outstanding malpractice cases that she knows about is not very reassuring. We live in a **litigious** society, and healthcare managers must understand professional liability and the need to be proactive in the creation and implementation of workable and effective incident reporting systems. Any unusual or potentially problematic event, medical or interpersonal, between a provider or staff member and a patient should be reported and reviewed by the medical director, and, as needed, by legal counsel. Pat needs to investigate whether CMG has an incident reporting system and whether it is being used effectively.

Informed consent
A legal document in all 50 states that constitutes an agreement for a proposed medical treatment or nontreatment, or for a proposed invasive procedure. It requires physicians to disclose the benefits, risks, and alternatives to the proposed treatment, nontreatment, or procedure. It is the method by which fully informed, rational persons may be involved in choices about their healthcare.

Tort
An intentional wrong that results in injury or harm. Breach of contract is a category of tort.

Litigious
Contentious and prone to become involved in lawsuits.

16.6 HEALTH ORGANIZATIONS AND EMPLOYEES

Health organizations are labor intensive and are often one of an area's largest employers. Health organizations employ a range of health professionals and other workers and are subject to the Fair Labor Standards Act of 1938, which ensures all employees access to a minimum wage, overtime, and equal pay for equal work and places restrictions on child labor.

The federal government has passed antidiscrimination laws to ensure equal employment opportunities to all qualified workers. The five primary statutes in this area are the following:

- ◆ Civil Rights Act of 1964: Bars discrimination based on race, color, religion, sex, national origin, or pregnancy

- ◆ Rehabilitation Act of 1973: Bars discrimination against handicapped persons

- ◆ Age Discrimination in Employment Act of 1975: Bars discrimination against persons over the age of 40

- ◆ Americans with Disabilities Act of 1990: Protects individuals with disabilities and requires employers to provide reasonable accommodations

- ◆ Family and Medical Leave Act of 1993: Requires employers with 50 or more employees to provide eligible employees up to 12 weeks per year of unpaid leave and continued health insurance coverage.

"Healthcare facilities are required to comply with all applicable Department of Health and Human Services regulations including but not limited to those pertaining to non-discrimination...their violation may result in the termination or suspension of or the refusal to grant or continue payment with federal funds" (Pozgar 1993, 473).

In the case study, Mark openly admits to refusing to consider job applicants who are overweight and unattractive. His comments about applicants with accents indicate that he may also have discriminated based on country of origin and perhaps race or color. And to make matters worse, it seems that Mark may have fired a nurse without collecting factual information about her alleged breach of confidentiality. Each of these is a serious offense in itself. Taken together, these incidents demonstrate a troubling pattern of unprincipled hiring and firing.

All employers are required to provide a safe working environment for their employees. The Occupational Safety and Health Act of 1970 was enacted to "assure, so far as possible, every working man and woman in the nation safe and healthful working conditions" (Pozgar 1993, 459). Potential exposure to blood, body fluids, wounds, waste matter, and the diseases that these substances can transmit make healthcare environments a safety challenge. Many health professionals are involved in patient ambulation, lifting, and transport, which present possible injuries. Finally, healthcare is rife with technologies, such as radiation, magnetic fields, and gases, that may endanger employees, particularly with repeated exposure.

An employee who is injured while performing work-related activities is generally eligible for **worker's compensation** insurance. Employers are required to provide worker's compensation as a benefit, and the law does not require proof that the injury was caused by the employer's negligence. Because worker's compensation is administered by each state, the scope of coverage varies widely from state to state. Health managers need to acquaint themselves with their state's specific worker's compensation laws and processes.

Pat Wheeler has good reason to be concerned about the attorney's visit in two days. Her discussion with Mark and Linda has revealed a number of events that may have triggered the lawsuit. But perhaps even more troubling is the fact that the prior administrator and the medical director seem unaware of the lawsuit and are quite cavalier about it. Regardless of the suit itself, Pat should begin a systematic review of all of CMG's policies and procedures. A manager's best protection from legal action is to prevent legal problems before they occur. Well-drafted and well-implemented policies and procedures are the first step.

Worker's compensation
Insurance overseen by the State for employees who are injured while performing work or work-related activities.

DISCUSSION QUESTIONS

➤ What does Pat need to do to prepare herself for her meeting with the attorney?

➤ To prove negligence in a malpractice suit, all four elements must be proven. Can you think of a situation where only three of the four elements are present?

➤ Informed consent seems relatively straightforward, but often it is not. What healthcare issues might make informed consent difficult to achieve?

EXERCISE 16.1 PROMISES, PROMISES, PROMISES

Casey Rosenburg had been hired four years earlier as the director of the HR department at Logan's New England Urgent Care Centers, a nationwide healthcare operation that had enjoyed financial success throughout its ten-year history. The number of patients had increased significantly, and industry analysts predicted growth and stock value increases.

Casey was optimistic about the urgent care centers. Patients were seen for annual checkups and for minor accidents and injuries. The healthcare clinical staff members took care of patients who had been hurt in everyday activities (e.g., an urgent care patient may have broken a bone playing on the local baseball team or tripping over the leash while walking the dog). They were known for their kind bedside manner and professional competence.

Casey's optimism was contagious. He constantly reminded the staff of Logan's tremendous potential. In fact, he had most of his employees convinced that high pay raises would come automatically if they just stayed with the company, maintained their level of competence, and kept treating the patients with kindness. "Just keep doing what you are doing" was one of his favorite counsels. Almost everyone liked Casey, and employee morale was high.

To even Casey's surprise, he was offered a position as the HR director for the Northwestern Urgent Care Centers. Melissa Kelly, who had been an assistant supervisor in the Southeastern Care Centers, was chosen to replace Casey. Melissa had established an excellent reputation in the Southeast. However, soon after Melissa took over the HR department, she discovered that Casey had made promises to the staff members that did not make sense to her. She knew she could not keep Casey's promises. Two staff members had been promised immediate raises. This was against Logan's policy and procedures. Raises were allocated annually for staff. Also, Casey had told all staff members to take vacation whenever they wanted to. Melissa could not understand how Casey planned to cover staffing with a promise like that one. Furthermore, Casey had not documented any of the hiring processes regarding the nursing staff that had been hired over the last two years. Melissa could not find any records of who applied, who was interviewed, and why the person hired was selected to work for Logan.

➤ What do you think of Casey's management skills?
➤ What do you think are the legal ramifications of Casey's management skills?
➤ What would you do if you were Melissa? Whom would you recommend she contact first?

EXERCISE 16.2   HIPAA AND THE PHONE CALL

Ruby Larusso called for an appointment with the Minnesota University Research Institute's legal counsel. She wanted to meet as soon as possible. The secretary informed her that she could come over right away, as the attorney did not have an appointment for the next hour. Ruby hurried from her office to the administration building where the attorney worked.

Ruby sat down in the attorney's office and quickly explained. "This morning, I received an angry phone call from Jake Lawson, a subject in the nutrition research project. It seems that Jake had told his boss at a fast-food restaurant that he was coming to the institute for doctors' appointments. When Jake's boss had asked him directly whether he was participating in a research project or coming for medical appointments, Jake had lied and answered that he was seeking medical attention. Jake called me because his boss fired him yesterday afternoon for lying to his supervisor. Jake said that he was going to sue because I had violated HIPAA regulations regarding his privacy rights."

Ruby further explained, "Yesterday, I received a phone call from someone inquiring whether patients were ever seen at the institute for medical appointments. I told the caller that the institute's sole purpose was research, and that any subject who might require medical attention would be referred to the appropriate clinic department at the university. I also said that we do not offer medical services to patients in the research institute. I did not disclose any information about Jake, nor did I discuss any of the current research studies with the caller. I think that caller might have been Jake's boss."

Ruby asked, "Am I in trouble? Did I violate HIPAA rules?"

➤ Do you think Ruby violated HIPAA rules? Why or why not?
➤ What action, if any, should Ruby and the attorney take at this time?

GLOSSARY

360 evaluation: A review process in which the supervisor, the employee, and staff members who work for the employee assess the work behavior and efforts of the employee.

Accommodating style: A conflict style involving low concern for one's own position and high concern for those of others.

Active listening: The process of paying close attention to a message so that it is sent and received accurately.

Activity-based budgeting: Creating a statement that focuses on the manager's allocating costs to each activity performed on behalf of the unit's responsibilities (such as patient care).

Adjourning: The final stage of teamwork, during which team members review outcomes and successes and individuals disengage from the team.

Aggressiveness: Behavior that is hostile and combative.

American College of Healthcare Executives (ACHE): An international professional society of more than 30,000 healthcare executives who lead hospitals, healthcare systems, and other healthcare organizations. ACHE has over 80 chapters that provide access to networking, education, and career development at the local level. ACHE publishes *Healthcare Executive, Journal of Healthcare Management*, and *Frontiers of Health Services Management*. ACHE also has its own publishing division, Health Administration Press, which published this text.

Antitrust legislation: Laws established to prevent the formation of monopolies or other business structures that prevent free trade or attempt to restrain commerce.

Assertiveness: Behavior that is positive and self-confident.

Assessment: (1) The act of measuring, appraising, and evaluating. (2) The act of determining the importance or value of some action, procedure, or structure.

Association of University Programs in Health Administration (AUPHA): An international association of more than 500 colleges and universities dedicated to improving health by promoting excellence in healthcare management education. AUPHA provides opportunities for member programs to learn from each other by influencing practice and by promoting the value of healthcare management education. AUPHA publishes *Journal of Healthcare Management Education*.

Authoritarian: A leadership style in which power is concentrated in the leader.

Autonomy: The state of being self-governing. The liberty to rule one's self, free of the controlling influence of others.

Avoidance style: A conflict style involving low concern for self and low concern for others. This style often presents itself as withdrawal or lack of cooperation.

Benchmarking: The process of comparing one organization or situation to similar organizations or situations using uniform measures.

Beneficence: An obligation to help and provide benefits to others.

Best of breed: An arrangement of IT systems that consists of many small, stand-alone, proprietary systems that function well for their dedicated departments, few of which actually interface with each other.

Best practices: Those actions, processes, and procedures used in a profession, discipline, or industry to achieve the highest outcomes.

Bias: A tendency to apply a negative or positive bent to a situation because of prejudicial thought.

Bribe: A gift bestowed to influence the receiver's conduct.

Budget: A statement that indicates financial administration for a set period of time.

Change process: The process whereby managed changed is envisioned and implemented (successfully or unsuccessfully) in an organization.

Change recipients: The staff members whose work behaviors may be affected by changes implemented.

Characteristic Leadership Model: A model that defines leadership as a collection of characteristics that all leaders share.

Clinical ethics: The overarching framework of morals and principles that underscores the provision of medical care to patients.

Competence: Having the skills and abilities to function in a particular way or in a specific situation.

Competencies: Specific areas in which leaders must have the skills and abilities to function adequately and appropriately.

Compromising style: A conflict style involving a reasonable level of concern for self and others. This approach is concerned about keeping both sides equal and actively searches for the middle ground, ensuring that one side doesn't give in more than the other.

Conceptual skills: A manager's comprehension of the overall organization and how it fits within the larger environment.

Confidentiality: Holding information as secret and private.

Control: (1) To guide or check; the act of accountability. (2) Ensuring that work is done correctly and in an appropriate timeframe.

Corporate citizenship: The duty of all businesses to provide a significant net positive contribution to the general good of customers, employees, the community, the environment, and the global community.

Criticality: The ultimate importance of an issue, the material effect upon the individuals, and the time pressure that might be involved in resolving the conflict.

Cultural adaptability: The willingness and ability to understand cultural differences and act upon that understanding for cooperative outcomes.

Cultural relativism: The understanding that another culture needs to be understood based on its own standards, beliefs, and traditions.

Dashboard report: A report that uses color to visually indicate whether the data meets the goal (green), is within a specified acceptable range outside of the goal (yellow), or falls to an unacceptable level (red).

Decision-making process: The thought and action that leads one to choose from a set of options.

Delegation: Assigning tasks to others; the ability to get work done through others.

Democratic: A leadership approach in which team members share governance.

Direct costs: Expenses associated with a specific activity provided by a unit.

Diversity: A list of characteristics that include race, ethnicity, educational level, socioeconomic status, culture, language, religion, disabilities, sexual orientation, age, and gender that indicates an individual's background.

Dominating style: A conflict style involving high concern for self and low concern for others; demanding and imposing one's will on others with little or no concern about the impact on the other party.

Downward communication: Communication that is primarily informational and initiated by the superior in the organization.

Dustbin delegation: Delegating only unpleasant, boring tasks the manager doesn't want to do.

EEOC: The Equal Employment Opportunity Commission, the U.S. government agency that enforces federal employment discrimination laws.

Effective: Having a definite or desired effect.

Effective communication: Communication in which the receiver receives and understands the message as the sender intended it.

Efficient: Productive with minimum waste or effort.

Emergency Medical Treatment and Active Labor Law Act of 1986 (EMTALA): Legislation created to address the perceived concern of "patient dumping"—the refusal to treat uninsured patients and instead transfer them to charitable hospitals without having been seen or having gotten any care. EMTALA requires hospitals and their affiliated physicians to screen and continue to treat emergency patients until they are stabilized or transferred.

Emotional intelligence (EQ): The ability to recognize one's own strengths and weaknesses, see the link between feelings and behaviors, manage impulsive feelings and distressing emotions, be attentive to emotional cues, show sensitivity and respect for others, be an open communicator, and be able to handle conflict, difficult people, and tense situations effectively.

Enterprise resource planning (ERP) system: An overarching IT system in which all users share a common database and operating system, with all systems being interoperable and all departments and functions sharing and using the same information.

Envisioning change: The process by which decision makers picture the future of operations.

Ethics: An internalized understanding of how one should behave.

Ethnocentrism: The tendency to judge aspects of other cultures based upon the standards, beliefs, and traditions of one's own culture.

Excess of revenue over expenses: In a nonprofit organization, the remaining cash after revenues minus expenses.

Expense: Costs incurred by a unit's actions.

Feedback: Critical assessment of information or action.

Fidelity: The quality of being faithful, accurate, and steadfast to an ideal, obligation, trust, or duty.

Fixed costs: Expenses that will be incurred regardless of volume.

Forming: The first stage of teamwork, during which members are given their charge or the purpose of the team.

Four Rights approach: Delegating by assigning the right task, the right person, the right communication, and the right feedback.

Functions Leadership Model: A model that defines leadership by the tasks and functions in which all leaders engage.

Functions of management: The basic responsibilities of a manager, which include planning, organizing, leading, and controlling.

Groupthink: Conformity to group values and ethics that can lead to negative outcomes.

Health Insurance Portability and Accountability Act's (HIPAA) Privacy Rule: Part of the Health Insurance Portability and Accountability Act that establishes safeguards to protect confidentiality and privacy and specifically identifies protected health information (PHI).

Implementing change: The process by which managers carry out the vision of the future of operations.

Incremental budgeting: Creating a financial statement that is increased or decreased according to previous expenditures for a set period of time.

Indirect costs: Expenses that are not associated with a specific unit activity.

Industrial Revolution: The shift from an agrarian-based economy to an industrial-based economy in Western countries in the eighteenth and nineteenth centuries. This shift resulted in changes to social and economic organization.

Informal power: The capacity to influence others without resorting to formal authority.

Informed consent: A legal document in all 50 states that constitutes an agreement for a proposed medical treatment or nontreatment, or for a proposed invasive procedure. It requires physicians to disclose the benefits, risks, and alternatives to the proposed treatment, nontreatment, or procedure. It is the method by which fully informed, rational persons may be involved in choices about their healthcare.

Integrity: Firm adherence to a code of ethics or to a moral code of behavior.

Interdisciplinary team: A group of people who represent different disciplines working together to accomplish a common goal.

Internalize: To incorporate values, beliefs, or norms as self-guiding principles.

Interpersonal skills: Those skills that are related to a manager's ability to work with people. Often called human skills or people skills.

IOMA: The Institute of Management and Administration, a professional organization for managers.

Job description: A document that clearly defines the tasks, duties, responsibilities, and performance standards associated with a position.

Joint Commission, The: A not-for-profit accrediting agency that assesses an organizations' ability to meet standards of performance in key healthcare operations.

Justice: Fairness. Ensuring that one is treated as one deserves.

Kickback: A form of bribery; the offering, giving, receiving, or soliciting of any item of value to influence the actions of another.

Laissez-faire: A "hands-off" leadership approach.

Lateral communication: Communication between staff members of the same status.

Lead: To be in charge of or responsible for people and/or tasks.

Leadership: The characteristic of guiding, directing, and assuming principal responsibility.

Level of authority: An employee's ability to carry out delegated tasks. Levels include the authority to search for information, the authority to provide recommendations, and the authority to fully implement a task.

Liability: Being in a position to likely incur an undesirable responsibility or obligation, usually monetary.

Litigious: Contentious and prone to become involved in lawsuits.

Malpractice: Injury or harm to a patient or customer directly caused by negligence, intentional tort, or breach of contract by a professional.

Managerial ethics: The overarching framework of morals and principles that underscores the oversight and leadership of others and of organizations.

Medical Group Management Association (MGMA): A professional association of medical group practice professionals with more than 21,500 members who lead and manage more than 13,500 organizations. Membership includes administrators, CEOs, physicians in management, board members, and office managers.

Multitasking: Doing more than one thing at a time.

Nonmaleficence: The quality of causing no injury or harm and committing no misconduct or wrongdoing.

Nonprogrammed decision: A decision for which there is no set procedure in place, and that must be resolved via rational thinking and action.

Nonverbal cues: In communication theory, the behaviors of persons who are interacting with one another. Body language, posture, and facial expressions may elaborate the message that is being sent or received.

Norming: The third stage of teamwork, during which team members agree upon working styles, conflict is reduced, and group cohesiveness emerges.

Open door management: Always working with your office door open to show that you are available to everyone all the time.

Organizational ethics: An overarching framework of morals and principles that underscores behavior in organizations.

Organizational fit: An employment candidate's qualification for the position advertised and ability to work well with others in the specific work environment.

Organizational politics: Exerting influence on individuals and on the outcomes of situations in an organization to meet one's own purposes, whether positive or negative.

Organize: To coordinate and carry out tasks.

Outcome: The end result, product, or conclusion to a process or event.

Performance evaluation: The process whereby the work behavior and efforts of employees is reviewed.

Performing: The fourth stage of teamwork, during which team members are engaged in the work and purpose of the team.

Plan: To devise or create a way to do or accomplish a defined task.

Positive duty: The duty of commission. The requirement to actively and intentionally engage in an action.

Power: The ability to enact one's own will based on status, rank, knowledge, level of education, reputation, or a combination of these and other factors.

Problem-solving style: A conflict style involving high concern for self and high concern for others. It searches for more than the middle ground and actively works toward finding the best possible outcome for all parties.

Process: A procedure or progression of activities performed to attain a specific outcome.

Profit: Total income or cash flow minus expenditures.

Protected health information (PHI): Information from which a specific person or patient can be identified and that relates to physical or mental health, the provision of healthcare, or the payment for healthcare.

Receiver: One who is given the message produced by the sender.

Refreezing: Stabilizing the forces that have brought about a newly implemented change so they become part of the organization.

Relationship conflict: Tension, animosity, and annoyance unrelated to the specific situation and interpersonal in nature.

Resistance to change: Change recipients' hesitation or refusal to comply with the vision of the future of operations and management attempts at carrying out the vision.

Resources: Physical or nonphysical features that are present or obtainable for use by an organization or individual.

Retention: The keeping of employees at an organization.

Revenue: Income produced by a unit's actions.

Risk: Uncertainty in an outcome.

Risk management: Systems, processes, and structures put in place to decrease the likelihood of adverse events.

Rolling budgeting: Creating a statement that indicates financial administration that is reviewed in a specified timeframe (monthly or quarterly) and updated.

Root cause analysis: The process of dissecting a positive or negative incident into its most basic segments and discovering the source of its characteristics and outcomes.

Running a morning dash: Spending an hour on the most important thing on your to-do list first thing each morning, even before checking your messages or e-mail.

Scientific management: The study of management activities based on theory and research.

Scientific method of inquiry: The formal process of research. Steps include observation and description, hypothesis formulation, data gathering, data analysis, and findings and conclusion discussion.

Sender: The producer of a message.

Sexual harassment: The illegal practice of unwelcome sexual behavior in the workplace.

Situationally appropriate: In a conflict, taking into account the power and criticality of the issue and each party's willingness to confront the other.

Socialization process: The process whereby people learn values, beliefs, and norms.

SS-LL dilemma: The basic conflict between short-term, more immediate costs and benefits and long-term, perhaps riskier, future payoffs.

Stakeholder: An individual, group, or entity that has an interest in organizational success.

Standards: Customary, appropriate, and acceptable criteria.

Statement of operations: A statement that shows the revenues, expenses, and income of an organization.

Storming: The second stage of teamwork, during which team members learn about one another. This stage is characterized by conflict and emotional issues that may inhibit a team's progress.

Structure: The environment and the set of conditions that exist. Structure is a necessary condition for quality to occur, but by itself it is insufficient to produce quality.

Task conflict: Disagreement about tasks, goals, methods, or desired outcomes.

Technical skills: Those skills that involve the specialized knowledge needed to get the work done.

Time inventory log: A tool that illustrates how time is used by briefly noting activities at regular intervals, perhaps each hour or half-hour, during the work day.

Tort: An intentional wrong that results in injury or harm. Breach of contract is a category of tort.

Train the trainer: The process of training one person or a small group of people, who then each train additional people, who then train more people, and so on.

Trust: Reliance on the truthfulness, honesty, and intentions of others.

Truth telling: A positive responsibility to provide accurate, complete, and honest information at all times as part of respect for persons.

Unfreezing: Reducing the forces that are keeping an organization in its current state.

Upward communication: Communication that allows supervisors to know about staff members' concerns, issues, or recommendations.

Variable costs: Expenses that will change as the volume changes.

Verbal cues: In communication theory, the tone and manner of the message sent and received.

Visionary: Having foresight, imagination, and the ability to form mental images of the future in a specific way.

Worker's compensation: Insurance overseen by the State for employees who are injured while performing work or work-related activities.

Zero-based budgeting: Creating a financial statement for a set period of time that requires each budget item to be justified according to the unit's goals.

REFERENCES

Academic Health Center Task Force. 1996. "Developing Health Care Teams." [Online article; retrieved 7/23/08.] www.ahc.umn.edu/tf/ihtd.html.

Adair, J. 2005. *How to Grow Leaders: The Seven Key Principles of Effective Leadership Development.* London: Kogan Page.

Adkins, B., and D. Caldwell. 2004. "Firm or Subgroup Culture: Where Does Fitting in Matter Most?" *Journal of Organizational Behavior* 25(8): 969–78.

Ales, B. 1995. "Mastering the Art of Delegation." *Nursing Management* 26 (8): 32A–33A.

Amason, A. C. 1996. "Distinguishing the Effects of Functional and Dysfunctional Conflict on Strategic Decision Making: Resolving a Paradox for Top Management Teams." *Academy of Management Journal* 39 (1): 123–48.

American College of Healthcare Executives (ACHE). 2006. "Impaired Healthcare Executives." [Online information; retrieved 6/26/07.] www.ache.org/policy/impaired.cfm.

———. 2005a. "Creating and Ethical Environment for Employees." [Online information; retrieved 6/26/07.] www.ache.org/policy/environ.cfm.

———. 2005b. "Statement on Diversity." [Online information; retrieved 6/26/07.] www.ache.org/policy/diversity.cfm.

———. 2004. "Health Information Confidentiality." [Online information; retrieved 6/26/07.] www.ache.org/policy/hiconf.cfm.

———. 2002. "Ethical Issues Related to Staff Shortages." [Online information; retrieved 6/26/07.] www.ache.org/policy/shortage.cfm.

American Medical Association. 2007. "Informed Consent." [Online information; retrieved 6/23/08.] www.ama-assn.org/ama/pub/category/4608.html.

American Psychological Association. 2006. "Advancing Colleague Assistance in Professional Psychology." [Online information; retrieved 6/26/07.] www.apa.org/practice/acca_monograph.pdf.

Amos, M., J. Hu, and C. Herrick. 2005. "The Impact of Team Building on Communication and Job Satisfaction of Nursing Staff." *Journal for Nurses in Staff Development* 21 (1): 10–16.

Anderson, L. 1993. "Teams: Group Processes, Success, and Barriers." *Journal of Nursing Administration* 23 (9): 15–19.

Andriof, J., and M. McIntosh (eds.). 2001. *Perspectives on Corporate Citizenship.* Sheffield, UK: Greenleaf Publishing.

Arndt, E. 1996. "Creating Organizational Vision in a Hospital Social Work Department: The Leitmotif for Continuous Change Management." *Administration in Social Work* 20 (4): 79–87.

Associated Press. 2006. "RadioShack Uses E-mail to Fire 400 Employees as Part of Planned Job Cuts." [Online article; retrieved 8/30/06.] www.ap.org.

Barczak, N. 1996. "How to Lead Effective Teams." *Critical Care Nursing Quarterly* 19 (1): 73–82.

Barnard, C. 1938. *The Functions of the Executive.* Cambridge: Harvard University Press.

Bartunek, J., D. Rousseau, J. Rudolph, and J. DePalma. 2006. "On the Receiving End: Sensemaking, Emotion, and Assessments of an Organizational Change Initiated by Others." *Journal of Applied Behavioral Science* 42 (2): 182–206.

Bastistella, R., J. Hill, S. Levey, and T. Weil. 2007. "Leadership Development in MHA Programs: A Response and Commentary." *Journal of Health Administration Education* 22 (3): 241–50.

Beer, M., R. Eisenstat, and B. Spector. 1990. "Why Change Programs Don't Produce Change." *Harvard Business Review* 68 (6): 158–66.

Birch, D. 2001. "Corporate Citizenship: Rethinking Business Beyond Corporate Social Responsibility." In *Perspectives on Corporate Citizenship*, edited by J. Andriof and M. McIntosh, 53–65. Sheffield, UK: Greenleaf Publishing.

Black, J. 2008. *The Toyota Way to Healthcare Excellence: Increase Efficiency and Improve Quality with Lean.* Chicago: Health Administration Press.

Blair, G. M. 1992. "Personal Time Management for Busy Managers." *Engineering Management Journal* 2 (1): 33–38.

Borrill, C., M. West, D. Shapiro, and A. Rees. 2000. "Team Working and Effectiveness in Health Care." *British Journal of Health Care Management* 6 (8): 364–71.

Bowen, D., G. Ledford, and B. Nathan. 1991. "Hiring for the Organization, Not the Job." *Academy of Management Executive* 5 (4): 35–51.

Buchmueller, T., and P. Feldstein. 1996. "Hospital Community Benefits Other Than Charity Care: Implications for Tax Exemption and Public Policy." *Hospital and Health Services Administration* 41 (4): 461–71.

Bucking, J. 2008. "Employee Terminations: 10 Must-Do Steps When Letting Someone Go." *Supervision* 69 (5): 11.

Burnes, B. 2007. "Kurt Lewin and the Harwood Studies: The Foundations of OD." *The Journal of Applied Behavioral Science* 43 (2): 213–31.

Byrne, Z. 2005. "Fairness Reduces the Negative Effects of Organizational Politics on Turnover Intentions, Citizenship Behavior and Job Performance." *Journal of Business and Psychology* 20 (2): 175–200.

Caesar, J. 1999. *The Gallic War.* Trans. C. Hammond. Oxford: Oxford University Press.

Callanan, G., and D. F. Perri. 2006. "Teaching Conflict Management Using a Scenario-Based Approach." *Journal of Education for Business* 81 (3): 131–39.

Caplan, G., A. Williams, B. Daly, and K. Abraham. 2004. "A Randomized Controlled Trial of Comprehensive Geriatric Assessment and Multidisciplinary Intervention After Discharge of Elderly from the Emergency Department—The DEED II Study." *Journal of the American Geriatric Society* 52 (9): 1417–23.

Caplow, T. 1983. *Managing an Organization.* New York: Holt, Rinehart, and Winston.

Carroll, J. S., and A.C. Edmondson. 2002. "Leading Organizational Learning in Health Care." *Quality and Safety in Health Care* 11 (1): 51–56.

Centers for Medicare & Medicaid Services. 2007. "EMTALA Overview." [Online information.] www.cms.hhs.gov/EMTALA.

Chatman, J. 1991. "Matching People and Organizations: Selection and Socialization in Public Accounting Firms." *Administrative Science Quarterly* 36 (3): 459–84.

Chou, H. W., and Y. J. Yeh. 2007. "Conflict, Conflict Management, and Performance in ERP Teams." *Social Behavior and Personality* 35 (8): 1035–48.

Clark, T. 1999 "Sharing the Importance of Attentive Listening Skills." *Journal of Management Education* 23 (2): 216–23.

Clinton, W. J. 1997. "Remarks by the President in Apology for Study Done in Tuskegee." [Online information; retrieved 12/22/08.] clinton4.nara.gov/textonly/New/Remarks/Fri/19970516-898.html.

Cohen, H., J. Feussner, M. Weinberger, R. Carnes, R. Hamdy, F. Hsieh, C. Phibbs, and P. Lavori. 2002. "A Controlled Trial of Inpatient and Outpatient Geriatric Evaluation and Management." *New England Journal of Medicine* 346 (12): 905–12.

Coile, R. C. 2002. *Futurescan 2002: A Forecast of Healthcare Trends.* Chicago: Health Administration Press.

Collins, J. C., and J. I. Porras. 1991. "Organizational Vision and Visionary Organizations." *California Management Review* 34 (1): 30–52.

Committee on Pediatric Workforce. 2000. "Enhancing the Racial and Ethnic Diversity of the Pediatric Workforce." *Pediatrics* 105 (1): 129–31.

Coser, L. 1971. *Masters of Sociological Thought.* New York; Harcourt Brace Jovanovich, Inc.

Council on Graduate Medical Education. 1998. "The Health Status of Minority Populations." In *Minorities in Medicine,* edited by U.S. Department of Health and Human Services, Health Resources and Services Administration, 7–13. Washington, DC: U.S. Department of Health and Human Services.

Couper, I. D. 2007. "The Impotance of Being Important: Reflections on Leadership." *Annals of Family Medicine* 5 (3): 261–62.

Couzins, M., and S. Beagrie. 2004. "How To . . . Build Effective Teams." *Personnel Today* Feb. 24: 29.

Covey, S. R. 1990. *The Seven Habits of Highly Effective People.* New York: Simon & Schuster.

Credit Suisse Learning. 2008. "Time Management: Fight Your Time Bandits." [Online article; retrieved 7/30/09.] emagazine.credit-suisse.com/app/article/index.cfm?aoid=27815&fuseaction=OpenArticle&lang=en.

Cropanzano, R. 2003. "Deontic Justice: The Role of Moral Principles in Workplace Fairness." *Journal of Organizational Behavior* 24 (8): 1019–24.

Culp, G., and A. Smith. 1997. "Six Steps to Effective Delegation." *Journal of Management in Engineering* 13 (1): 30–31.

Curtis, E., and H. Nicholl 2004. "Delegation: A Key Function of Nursing." *Nursing Management* 11(4): 26–31.

Daft, R. L. 1991. *Management.* Chicago: Dryden Press.

Davies, E. 1996. "How Violence at Work Can Hit Employees Hard." *People Management* 2: 50–53.

Deal, J. J., and D. W. Prince. 2003. *Developing Cultural Adaptability: How to Work Across Differences.* Greensboro, NC: Center for Creative Leadership.

DeDreu, C. K., and L. R. Weingart. 2003. "Task Versus Relationship Conflict, Team Performance, and Team Member Satisfaction: A Meta-Analysis." *Journal of Applied Psychology* 88 (4): 741–49.

Descartes, R. 1637. *Discourse on Method and the Meditations.* Trans. F. E. Sutcliffe. London: Penguin.

Dessler, G. 2009. *Fundamentals of Human Resource Management.* Upper Saddle River, NJ: Prentice Hall.

Donabedian, A. 1966. "Evaluating the Quality of Medical Care." *Milbank Memorial Fund Quarterly* 44 (3): 166–202.

Donoghue, C. and N. Castle. 2007. "Organizational and Environmental Effects on Voluntary and Involuntary Turnover." *Health Care Management Review* 32 (4): 360–69.

Drucker, P. 2001. *The Essential Drucker.* New York: HarperCollins.

———.1988. "Leadership: More Doing than Dash." *The Wall Street Journal*, January 6.

———. 1974. *Management: Tasks, Responsibilities, Practices.* New York: Harper & Row.

———. 1967. *The Effective Executive.* New York: HarperCollins.

Dunn, R. 2007. *Haimann's Healthcare Management*, 8th ed. Chicago: Health Administration Press.

Durutta, N. 2006. "The Corporate Communicator: A Senior-Level Strategist." In *The IABC Handbook of Organizational Communication*, edited by T. L. Gillis. San Francisco: Jossey-Bass.

Dye, C., and A. N. Garman. 2006. *Exceptional Leadership: 16 Critical Competencies for Healthcare Executives.* Chicago: Health Administration Press.

Encyclopedia of Surgery. 2007. "Informed Consent." [Online article, retrieved 6/23/08.] www.surgeryencyclopedia.com/Fi-La/Informed-Consent.html.

Equal Employment Opportunity Commission (EEOC). 2008. "Sexual Harrassment." [Online article; retrieved 6/23/08.] www.eeoc.gov/types/sexual_harassment.html.

Ettinger, W. 2001. "Six Sigma: Adapting GE's Lessons to Healthcare." *Trustee* 54 (8): 10–16.

Fayol, H. 1916. *Industrial and General Administration.* Paris: Dunod.

Fisher, R., W. Ury, and B. Patton. 1991. *Getting to Yes: Negotiating Agreement Without Giving In.* New York: Penguin Books.

Flaherty, J. 1999. *Peter Drucker: Shaping the Managerial Mind.* San Francisco: Jossey-Bass.

Follett, M. 1941. *Dynamic Administration: The Collected Papers of Mary Parker Follett,* edited by H. Metcalf and L. Urwick. New York: Harper's.

Fottler, M. D. 2001. "Job Analysis and Job Design." In *Human Resources in Healthcare: Managing for Success,* edited by B. J. Fried and J. A. Johnson, 87–115. Chicago: Health Administration Press.

Gardenswartz, L. and A. Rowe. 2009. "The Effective Management of Cultural Diversity." In *Contemporary Leadership and Intercultural Competence.* edited by M. A. Moodian, 35–43. Los Angeles: Sage.

Garman, A., P. Butler, and L. Brinkmeyer. 2006. "Leadership." *Journal of Healthcare Management* 61 (6): 360–64.

Garner, B. A. (ed.). 2004. *Black's Law Dictionary,* 8th ed. St. Paul, MN: West Group.

Gerard, M. B. 2008. "Personal Time Management for Busy Managers: The 'Eff' Words." [Online article; retrieved 4/22/09.] www.see.ed.ac.uk/~gerard/Management/art2.html.

Gering, J., and J. Conner. 2002. "A Strategic Approach to Employee Retention." *Healthcare Financial Management* 56 (11): 40–44.

Giganti, E. 2004. "Organization Ethics Is 'Systems Thinking.'" *Health Progress* 85 (3): 10–11.

Gilbert, D. R. 1991. "Respect for Persons, Management Theory, and Business Ethics." In *Business Ethics: The State of the Art,* edited by R. E. Freeman, 111–20. Oxford, UK: Oxford University Press.

Gilbreth, F. 1916. "Motion Study in Surgery." *Canadian Journal of Medicine and Surgery* 40: 22–31.

———. 1914. "Scientific Management in the Hopsital." *Modern Hospital* 3: 321–24.

Goffman, E. 1959. *The Presentation of Self in Everyday Life*. Garden City, NJ: Doubleday.

Gratto Liebler, J., and C. R. McConnell. 2008. *Management Skills for the New Heath Care Supervisor*, 5th ed. Boston: Jones and Bartlett Publishers.

Greenleaf, R. K. 1977. *Servant Leadership: A Journey into the Nature of Legitimate Power and Greatness*. New York: Paulist Press.

Griffith, J. and K. White. 2007. *The Well-Managed Healthcare Organization*, 6th ed. Chicago: Health Administration Press.

Hantsen, R., and M. Washburn. 1992. "How to Plan What to Delegate." *American Journal of Nursing* 92 (4): 71–72.

Harmon, S., S. Brallier, and G. Brown. 2002. "Organizational and Team Context." In *Team Performance in Health Care*, edited by G. Heinemann and A. Zeiss, 57–70. New York: Kluwer Academic/Plenum Publishers.

Harris, G. 2007. "If Your Only Tool Is a Hammer, Any Issue Will Look Like a Nail: Building Conflict Resolution and Mediation Capacity in South African Universities." *Higher Education* 55 (1): 93–101.

Harris, P. R., R. T. Moran, and S. V. Moran. 2004. *Managing Cultural Differences: Global Leadership for the Twenty-First Century*, 6th ed. Oxford, UK: Elsevier-Butterworth-Heinemann.

Hartman, L. P. 1998. *Perspectives in Business Ethics*. Chicago: Irwin McGraw-Hill.

Harvard Business School. 2005. *Time Management: Increase Your Personal Productivity and Effectiveness*. Boston: Harvard Business School Press.

Hastings, D. A., G. M. Luce, and N. A. Wynstra. 1995. *Fundamentals of Health Law*. Washington, DC: National Health Lawyers Association.

Health West, Inc. 2007. "Mission Statement." [Online information; retrieved 8/8/08.] www.healthwestinc.org.

Healthlinks. 2007. "Frequently Asked Questions about the Emergency Medical Treatment and Active Labor Act (EMTALA)." [Online information; retrieved 4/23/09.] www.emtala.com/faq.htm.

Heinemann, G. 2002. "Teams in Health Care Settings: Assessment and Development." In *Team Performance in Health Care*, edited by G. Heinemann and A. Zeiss, 3–17. New York: Kluwer Academic/Plenum Publishers.

Heinemann, G. D., M. P. Farrell, and M. H. Schmitt. 1994. "Groupthink Theory and Research: Implications for Decision Making in Geriatric Health Care Teams." *Educational Gerontology* 20(1): 71–85.

Heller, J. 1972. "Syphilis Victims in the U.S. Study Went Untreated for 40 Years." *New York Times,* July 26.

Hellriegel, D., and J. Slocum. 2003. *Organizational Behavior*, 10th ed. Cincinnati, OH: Southwestern College Publishing.

Hensel, J. 2000. "Reading the Signs." *Occupational Health and Safety* 69 (9): 20.

Hinckley, R. C. 2002. "28 Words to Redefine Corporate Duties: The Proposal for Corporate Citizenship." *Multinational Monitor* 23 (7): 18–20.

Hoffman, B. J. and D. J. Woehr. 2006. "A Quantitative Review of the Relationship Between Person-Organization Fit and Behavioral Outcomes." *Journal of Vocational Behavior* 68 (3): 389–99.

Huse, E. G. 1975. *Organization Development and Change*. St. Paul, MN: West Publishing.

Institute of Medicine, Committee on Quality of Health Care in America. 2001. *Crossing the Quality Chasm: A New Health System for the 21ˢᵗ Century*. Washington, DC: National Academies Press.

———. Committee on Quality of Health Care in America. 2000. *To Err Is Human: Building a Safer Health System*. Washington, DC: National Academies Press.

Isenberg, S. F. 2007. "Double-Dose Decline." *ENT: Ear, Nose and Throat Journal* 86 (11): 670.

Janus, I. 1972. *Victims of Groupthink: A Psychological Study of Foreign-Policy Decisions and Fiascos*. Boston: Houghton Mifflin.

Jehn, K. A., and E. A. Mannix. 2001. "The Dynamic Nature of Conflict: A Longitudinal Study of Intragroup Conflict and Group Performance." *Academy of Management Journal* 44 (2): 238–51.

Jick, T. D. 1993. *Managing Change*. Homewood, IL: Irwin.

Joint Commission, The. 2008. [Online information; retrieved 6/30/08.] http://www.jointcommission.org.

————. 1995. *Comprehensive Accreditation Manual for Hospitals*. Oakbrook Terrace, IL: The Joint Commission.

Jones, J. H. 1981. *Bad Blood: The Tuskegee Syphilis Experiment: A Tragedy of Race and Medicine*. New York: Free Press.

Kacmar, K. M., and R. A. Baron. 1999. "Organizational Politics: The State of the Field, Links to Related Processes, and an Agenda for Future Research." In *Research in Personnel and Human Resources Management*, edited by G. R. Ferris, 1–39. Greenwich, CT: JAI Press.

Kahn, R. A. 2004. "Records Management and Compliance: Making the Connection." *Information Management Journal* 38 (3): 28–36.

Kanter, R. M. 2001. *Evolve: Succeeding in the Digital Culture of Tomorrow*. Boston: Harvard Business Publisher.

Kanter, R. M., B. A. Stein, and T. D. Jick. 1992. *The Challenge of Organizational Change*. New York: Free Press.

Katz, R. 1974. "Skills of an Effective Administrator." *Harvard Business Review* 52 (5): 90–102.

Kitson, A., and A. R. Campbell. 1996. *The Ethical Organization: Ethical Theory and Corporate Behavior*. Basingstoke, UK: Macmillan Press.

Kohler Company. 2009. Mission statement. Personal communication, January 12.

Konig, C. J., and M. Kleinmann. 2007. "Time Management Problems and Discounted Utility." *The Journal of Psychology* 141 (3): 321–34.

Kopeikina, L. 2006. "The Elements of a Clear Decision." *MIT Sloan Management Review* 47 (2): 19–20.

Kourdi, J. 1999. *Successful Delegation*. London: Hodder and Stoughton.

Kristof, A. L. 1996. "Person-Organization Fit: An Integrative Review of Its Conceptualizations, Measurement, and Implications." *Personnel Psychology* 49 (1): 1–49.

Kulesher, R. R., and M. G. Wilder. 2008. "The Impact of PPS on Hospital-Sponsored Post-Acute Services: A Case Study of Delaware Medicare Providers." *Journal of Healthcare Management* 53 (1): 54–66.

Lemieux-Charles, L., and W. McGuire. 2006. "What Do We Know About Health Care Team Effectiveness? A Review of the Literature." *Medical Care Research and Review* 63(3): 263–300.

Lewin, K. 1947. "Frontiers in Group Dynamics." *Human Relations* 1 (1): 5–41.

Lewis, B. J. 2000. "Management by Delegation." *Journal of Management in Engineering* 16 (2): 21.

Lewis, L. K. 2007. "An Organizational Stakeholder Model of Change Implementation Communication." *Communication Theory* 17 (2): 176–204.

Lynn, J., M. A. Baily, M. Bottrell, B. Jennings, R. J. Levine, F. Davidoff, D. Casarett, J. Corrigan, E. Fox, M. K. Wynia, G. J. Agich, M. O'Kane, T. Speroff, P. Schyve, P. Batalden, S. Tunis, N. Berlinger, L. Cronenwett, J. M. Fitznaurice, N. N. Dubler, and B. James. 2007. "The Ethics of Using Quality Improvement Methods in Health Care." *Annals of Internal Medicine* 146 (9): 666–73.

Margolis, J. D. 2001. "Responsibility in Organizational Context." *Business Ethics Quarterly* 11 (3): 431–54.

Marquis, B. L., and C. J. Huston. 2000. *Leadership Roles and Management Functions in Nursing.* New York: Lippincott, Williams & Wilkins.

McDonald, A., and T. Leyhane. 2005. "Drill Down with Root Cause Analysis: Know the Source of the Spark While Protecting Yourself from the Fire." *Nursing Management* 36 (1): 26–32.

McGinnis, S. K., L. D. Pumphrey, K. J. Trimmer, and C. Wiggins. 2004. "A Case Study in IT Innovation in a Small, Rural Community Hospital." *Research in Healthcare Financial Management* 9 (10): 9–21.

McIlwain, J. C. 2006. "A Review: A Decade of Clinical Risk Management and Risk Tools." *Clinician in Management* 14 (4): 189–99.

Medical Group Management Association. 2009. MGMA Diversity Statement. [Online information; retrieved 8/5/09.] www.mgma.com/about/default.aspx?id=200.

Miles, R. H. 1980. *Macro Organizational Behavior.* Glenview, IL: Scott Foresman.

Mintzberg, H. 1983. *Power in and Around Organizations.* Englewood Cliffs, NJ: Prentice-Hall.

Mott, W. J. 2003. "Developing a Culturally Competent Workforce: A Diversity Program in Progress." *Journal of Healthcare Management* 48 (5): 337–42.

Nash, L. 1989. "Ethics Without the Sermon." In *Ethics in Practice: Managing the Moral Corporation,* edited by K. R. Andrews, 243–56. Boston: Harvard Business Review.

National Center for Healthcare Leadership (NCHL). 2004. [Online information; retrieved 8/4/08.] www.nchl.org/ns/documents/documents.asp.

O'Reilly, C. A., J. A. Chatman, and D. F. Caldwell. 1991. "People and Organizational Culture: A Profile Comparison Approach to Assessing Person-Organization Fit." *Academy of Management Journal* 34 (3): 963–75.

Palmer, J. K., and J. M. Loveland. 2008. "The Influence of Group Discussion on Performance Judgments: Rating Accuracy, Contrast Effects, and Halo." *Journal of Psychology* 142 (2): 117–30.

Parsons, P. J. 2001 *Beyond Persuasion: The Healthcare Manager's Guide to Strategic Communication.* Chicago: Health Administration Press.

Parsons, T. 1951. *The Social System.* Glencoe, IL: Free Press.

Peer, K. S., and J. S. Rakich. 1999. "Ethical Decision Making in Healthcare Management." *Hospital Topics* 77 (4): 7–13.

Pelote, V., and L. Route. 2007. *Masterpieces in Healthcare Leadership: Cases and Analysis for Best Practice.* Sudbury, MA: Jones and Bartlett.

Pendry, L. F., D. M. Driscoll, and S. C. Field. 2007. "Diversity Training: Putting Theory into Practice." *Journal of Occupational and Organizational Psychology* 80 (1): 27–50.

Portny, S. E. 2002. "The Delegation Dilemma: When Do You Let Go?" *Information Management Journal* 36 (2): 60–64.

Posavac, E. J., and R. G. Carey. 1997. *Program Evaluation: Methods and Case Studies*, 5th ed. Upper Saddle River, NJ: Prentice Hall.

Pozgar, G. D. 1993. *Legal Aspects of Health Care Administration.* Gaithersburg, MD: Aspen.

Rachlin, H., A. Raineri, and D. Cross. 1991. "Subjective Probability and Delay." *Journal of the Experimental Analysis of Behavior* 55 (2): 233–44.

Rahim, M. A. 2002. "Toward a Theory of Managing Organizational Conflict." *International Journal of Conflict Management* 13 (3): 206–35.

———. 2001. *Managing Conflict in Organizations.* 3rd ed. Westport, CT: Quorum Books.

Rawls, J. 2001. *Justice as Fairness: A Restatement.* Cambridge, MA: Belknap Press.

Reutter, L., P. A. Field, I. E. Campbell, and R. Day, R. 1997. "Socialization into Nursing: Nursing Students as Learners." *Journal of Nursing Education* 36 (4): 149–55.

Robbins, S. 2000. *Managing Today!* 2nd ed. Upper Saddle River, NJ: Prentice Hall.

Rocchiccioli, J. T., and M. S. Tilbury. 1998. *Clinical Leadership in Nursing.* Philadelphia, PA: WB Saunders.

Rooney, J., and L. Vanden Heuvel. 2004. "Root Cause Analysis for Beginners." *Quality Progress* 37 (7): 45–53.

Ross, A., F. J. Wenzel, and J. W. Mitlyng. 2002. *Leadership for the Future: Core Competencies in Healthcare.* Chicago: Health Administration Press.

Rue, L. W., and L. L. Byars. 2004. *Supervision: Key Link to Productivity.* Boston: McGraw-Hill Irwin.

Ruusuvuori, J. 2001. "Looking Means Listening: Coordinating Displays of Engagement in Doctor-Patient Interaction." *Social Science and Medicine* 52 (7): 1093–1108.

Shannon, C. E., and W. Weaver. 1949. *The Mathematical Theory of Communication.* Urbana, IL: University of Illinois Press.

Shi, L. 2007. *Managing Human Resources in Health Care Organizations.* Boston: Jones and Bartlett.

Shi, L., and D. Singh. 2001. *Delivering Health Care in America.* Gaithersburg, MD: Aspen.

Showalter, J. S. 2007. *The Law of Healthcare Administration,* 5th ed. Chicago: Health Administration Press.

Simon, H. A. 1977. *The New Science of Management Decision.* Englewood Cliffs, NJ: Prentice-Hall.

Solansky, S. 2008. "Leadership Style and Team Processes in Self-Managed Teams." *Journal of Leadership and Organizational Studies* 14 (4): 332–41.

Sportsman, S. 2007. "The Human Resources Functions in Hospitals." In *Managing Human Resources in Health Care Organizations,* edited by L. Shi, 185–223. Boston: Jones and Bartlett.

St. James, E. 2001. *Simplify Your Work Life.* New York: Hyperion.

Sternberg, S. 2002. "For City's Hospital, Help Is Needed 'in a Hurry.'" *USAToday.* [Online article; retrieved 6/20/07.] www.usatoday.com/news/nation/2005-09-01-coverkatrina _x.htm.

Stevens, R. 1971. *American Medicine and the Public Interest.* New Haven, CT: Yale University Press.

Sumner, W. G. 1906. *Folkways.* Repr., New York: Dover, 1959.

Sutton, R. I. 2002. *Weird Ideas That Work.* New York: Free Press.

Sutton, R. I., and R. L. Kahn. 1986. "Prediction, Understanding, and Control as Antidotes to Organizational Stress." In *Handbook of Organizational Behavior,* edited by J. W. Lorsch, 272–85. Englewood Cliffs, NJ: Prentice-Hall.

Taylor, F. 1911. *The Principles of Scientific Management*. New York: Harper Bros.

Thompson, J. 2007. "The Strategic Management of Human Resources." In *Introduction to Health Care Management*, ed. S. B. Buchbinder and N. H. Shanks, 265–301. Boston: Jones and Bartlett.

Trapani, G. 2006. *Lifehacker: 88 Tech Tricks to Turbocharge Your Day*. New York: John Wiley and Sons.

Trunk, P. 2008. "10 Tips for Time Management in a Multitasking World." [Online article, retrieved 2/8/08.] blog.penelopetrunk.com/2006/12/10/10-tips-for-time-management-in-a-multitasking-world/.

Tuckman, B. 1965. "Developmental Sequences in Small Groups." *Psychological Bulletin* 63: 384–99.

Tuckman, B. and M. Jensen. 1977. "Stages of Small Group Development Revisited." *Group and Organizational Studies* 2 (4): 419–27.

United Press International. 2002. "Enron Whistle-Blower Testifies to Congress." [Online article; retrieved 8/5/09.] www.newsmax.com/archives/articles/2002/2/14/165328.shtml.

Universty of Texas M.D. Anderson Cancer Center. 2009. "Mission, Vision, and Core Values." [Online information; retrieved 1/13/09.] www.mdanderson.org/about_mda/who_we_are/display.cfm?id=D78111CE-7845-11D4-AEC300508BDCCE3A&method=displayFull.

University of Virginia Health System. 2006. "Mission, Vision, and Values." [Online information, retrieved 8/9/08.] www.healthsystem.virginia.edu/toplevel/why-choose/overview/mission/home.cfm.

U.S. Census Bureau. 2001. *Statistical Abstract of the United States 2001*. Washington, DC: U.S. Census Bureaus.

U.S. Department of Health and Human Services. 2002. "20 Tips to Help Prevent Medical Errors in Children." [Online article; retrieved 6/28/07.] www.ahrq.gov/consumer/20tips.htm.

Vaccaro, P. J. 2003. "Forget About Time Management." *Family Practice Management* 10 (5): 82.

Valle, M. 2006. "The Power of Politics: Why Leaders Need to Learn the Art of Influence." *Leadership in Action* 26 (2): 8–12.

Valle, M., and L. A. Witt. 2001. "The Moderating Effect of Teamwork Perceptions on the Organizational Politics–Job Satisfaction Relationship." *Journal of Social Psychology* 141 (3): 379–88.

Vogel, S. 2008. "Trying Some Disney Attitude to Help Cure Walter Reed." *Washington Post*, February 25.

Voltaire, F. 1762. *Candide*. Trans. T. Cuffe. New York: Penguin, 2005.

Von Bergen, C. W., B. Soper, and T. Foster. 2002. "Unintended Negative Effects of Diversity Management." *Public Personnel Management* 31 (2): 239–51.

Waddock, S., and N. Smith. 2000. "Corporate Responsibility Audits: Doing Well by Doing Good." *MIT Sloan Management Review* 41: 75–83.

Wager, K. A., F. W. Lee, and J. P. Glaser. 2005. *Managing Health Care Information Systems*. San Francisco: Jossey-Bass.

Warburton, J., M. Shapiro, A. Buckley, and Y. van Gellecum. 2004. "A Nice Thing to Do but Is It Critical for Business?" *Australian Journal of Social Issues* 39 (2): 117–27.

Weisman, D., D. Gordon, S. Cassard, M. Bergner, and R. Wong. 1993. "The Effects of Unit Self-Management on Hospital Nurses' Work Process, Work, Satisfaction, and Retention." *Medical Care* 31 (5): 381–93.

Wentling, R. M., and N. Palma-Rivas. 1999. "Components of Effective Diversity Training Programs." *International Journal of Training and Development* 3 (3): 215–26.

Wenzel, F. J., and J. M. Wenzel. 2005. *Fundamentals of Physician Practice Management*. Chicago: Health Administration Press.

Werhane, P. H. 1985. *Persons, Rights, and Corporations*. Englewood Cliffs, NJ: Prentice-Hall.

Whitman, M. V., and J. A. Davis. 2008. "Implementing Cultural and Linguistic Competence in Healthcare Management Curriculum." *Journal of Health Administration Education* 25 (1): 109–25.

Whitworth, A. 2005. "The Politics of Virtual Learning Environments: Environmental Change, Conflict, and E-learning." *British Journal of Educational Technology* 36 (4): 685–91.

Whitworth, B. 2006. "The Corporate Communicator: A Senior-Level Strategist." In *The IABC Handbook of Organizational Communication*, edited by T. L. Gillis, 205–14. San Francisco: Jossey-Bass.

Wiggins, C. 2000. "Healthcare Managers at Work: Be Careful Out There!" *Hospital Topics* 78 (4): 21–25.

Wiggins, C., J. Beachboard, K. Trimmer, and L. Pumphrey. 2006. "Entrepreneurial IT Governance: Electronic Medical Records in Rural Healthcare." *International Journal of Healthcare Information Systems and Informatics* 1(4): 40–53.

Wiggins, C., and S. Y. Bowman. 2000. "Career Success and Life Satisfaction for Female and Male Healthcare Managers." *Hospital Topics* 78(3): 5–10.

Wiggins, C., L. Hatzenbuehler, and T. Peterson 2008."Hospital Missions and the Education of Our Future Health Care Workforce." *Journal of Allied Health* 37 (3): 132–36.

Winkler, E. C., and R. L. Gruen. 2005. "First Principles: Substantive Ethics for Healthcare Organizations." *Journal of Healthcare Management* 50 (2): 109–19.

Witt, L. A, M. C. Andrews, and K. M. Kacmar. 2000. "The Role of Participative Decision Making in the Organizational Politics–Job Satisfaction Relationship." *Human Relations* 53(3): 341–57.

Wynia, M. K., S. R. Latham, and A. C. Kao. 1999. "Medical Professionalism in Society." *New England Journal of Medicine* 341 (21): 1612–16.

Zuckerman, H., W. Dowling, and M. Richardson, M. 2000. "The Managerial Role." In *Health Care Management: Organization Design and Behavior*, 4th ed., edited by S. Shortell and A. Kaluzny, 34–60. Albany, NY: Delmar.

INDEX

ABOUT THE AUTHORS

Leigh W. Cellucci, PhD, earned an undergraduate degree in sociology from the College of Charleston in Charleston, South Carolina; a master's in sociology from the College of William and Mary in Williamsburg, Virginia; a PhD in sociology from the University of Virginia in Charlottesville, Virginia; and an MBA from Idaho State University in Pocatello, Idaho. She has served as faculty at Francis Marion University in Florence, South Carolina. She is currently associate professor and chair of the Health Care Administration Department at Idaho State University.

Carla Wiggins, PhD, earned her undergraduate degree in health services administration from Ithaca College in Ithaca, New York, and her doctoral degree in health services research, policy, and administration from the University of Minnesota in Minneapolis. She has served as faculty at Ithaca College; Franklin University in Columbus, Ohio; and Idaho State University in Pocatello, Idaho. She is currently on the faculty of the University of Wisconsin at Milwaukee. She is a frequent author and speaker both locally and nationally.